Sara Wells

Horizons of Healing
Complementary Arcturian Medicine

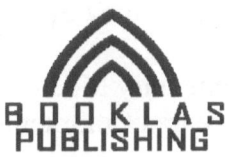

Original Title: Horizons of Healing – Complementary Arcturian Medicine

Copyright © 2025, published by Luiz Antonio dos Santos ME.

This book is a non-fiction work that explores practices and concepts within the field of integrative and cosmic healing. Through a comprehensive approach, the author offers practical tools to achieve emotional balance, spiritual alignment, and holistic health by bridging ancestral wisdom, integrative medicine, and Arcturian knowledge.

1st Edition
Production Team
Author: Sara Wells
Editor: Luiz Santos
Cover: Studios Booklas / **Marian Foster**
Consultant: Ethan Hargrove
Researchers: Livia Croft, **Jonathan Mendes**, **Priya Arora**
Layout: Carlos DeWitt
Translation: Angela Moretti

Publication and Identification
Horizons of Healing – Complementary Arcturian Medicine
Booklas, 2025
Categories: Integrative Medicine / Spiritual Healing / Cosmic Wisdom
DDC: 615.852 (Complementary Medicine and Healing)
CDU: 615.89 (Alternative and Complementary Therapies)

All rights reserved to:
Luiz Antonio dos Santos ME / Booklas Publishing

No part of this book may be reproduced, stored in a retrieval system, or transmitted by any means — electronic, mechanical, photocopying, recording, or otherwise — without prior written permission from the copyright holder.

Summary

Index Sistematic 5
Prologue 10
Chapter 1 Integrative Medicine 14
Chapter 2 The Arcturian Civilization and Its Wisdom 23
Chapter 3 Energy and Healing 31
Chapter 4 The Chakras and Health 39
Chapter 5 The Connection with Nature 47
Chapter 6 Arcturian Meditation and Visualization 55
Chapter 7 Arcturian Energy Healing 64
Chapter 8 Using Crystals and Sacred Geometry 72
Chapter 9 Arcturian Aromatherapy 80
Chapter 10 Arcturian Breathing Techniques 88
Chapter 11 Arcturian Hands-On Healing 96
Chapter 12 Arcturian Psychic Surgery 105
Chapter 13 Astral Travel and Distance Healing 113
Chapter 14 Energy Cleansing and Protection 122
Chapter 15 DNA Rebalancing 131
Chapter 16 Treatment of Chronic Diseases 139
Chapter 17 Mental and Emotional Health 147
Chapter 18 Pain Treatment 156
Chapter 19 Women's Health 164
Chapter 20 Child Health 172
Chapter 21 The Importance of Mindful Eating 180
Chapter 22 Physical Exercises and Movement 188

Chapter 23 The Power of Restorative Sleep 196
Chapter 24 The Healing of the Soul and Life Purpose 204
Chapter 25 Integration with Conventional Medicine................ 212
Chapter 26 The Expansion of Consciousness and Planetary Healing 220
Chapter 27 The Ethics of Arcturian Medicine in Practice 228
Chapter 28 The Training of Arcturian Therapists..................... 237
Chapter 29 The Future of Arcturian Medicine.......................... 244
Epilogue 253

Index Sistematic

Chapter 1: Integrative Medicine - Explores the principles of integrative medicine, highlighting the interconnection between the physical, emotional, mental, and spiritual dimensions of health.

Chapter 2: The Arcturian Civilization and Its Wisdom - Introduces the Arcturian civilization, their advanced technologies, and their integrated approach to healing, emphasizing the connection between science, spirituality, and medicine.

Chapter 3: Energy and Healing - Explores the concept of energy as the foundation of life and health, discussing the role of chakras, meridians, and subtle energy fields in the healing process.

Chapter 4: The Chakras and Health - Delves into the seven main chakras, their functions, and their influence on physical, emotional, mental, and spiritual well-being, offering practices for harmonizing these energy centers.

Chapter 5: The Connection with Nature - Explores the ancestral and inseparable relationship between humans and nature, highlighting the healing power of natural elements, medicinal plants, crystals, water, air, and sunlight.

Chapter 6: Arcturian Meditation and Visualization - Introduces the practice of Arcturian meditation and visualization as a spiritual technology for healing, reprogramming limiting patterns, and expanding consciousness.

Chapter 7: Arcturian Energy Healing - Presents Arcturian energy healing as a practice that combines vibrational science and spiritual understanding, using conscious intention, creative visualization, and advanced techniques to restore harmony and balance.

Chapter 8: Using Crystals and Sacred Geometry - Explores the use of crystals and sacred geometry in Arcturian medicine, highlighting their ability to amplify healing energies and restore vibrational coherence.

Chapter 9: Arcturian Aromatherapy - Introduces Arcturian aromatherapy, where essential oils are seen as olfactory light codes that promote vibrational harmonization and healing.

Chapter 10: Arcturian Breathing Techniques - Explores Arcturian breathing techniques as a way to access expanded states of consciousness, harmonize energy flows, and reconnect with the universal web of energy and information.

Chapter 11: Arcturian Hands-On Healing - Presents Arcturian hands-on healing as a practice that channels higher frequencies to restore balance and promote self-recognition and reconnection with the primordial essence.

Chapter 12: Arcturian Psychic Surgery - Introduces Arcturian psychic surgery, a spiritual technology that acts directly on the vibrational layers of the energy body to restore harmony and promote healing.

Chapter 13: Astral Travel and Distance Healing - Explores astral travel and distance healing as interdimensional practices that allow access to other planes of existence and the ability to act directly on energy structures regardless of physical or temporal location.

Chapter 14: Energy Cleansing and Protection - Discusses the importance of energy cleansing and protection for maintaining vibrational integrity, offering techniques to remove negative energies and strengthen the subtle bodies.

Chapter 15: DNA Rebalancing - Explores DNA rebalancing as a way to access and activate hidden layers of the human genetic code, promoting physical healing, emotional release, and the activation of dormant potentials.

Chapter 16: Treatment of Chronic Diseases - Presents the Arcturian approach to treating chronic diseases, emphasizing the identification of root causes, the integration of conventional and complementary therapies, and the importance of diet and lifestyle.

Chapter 17: Mental and Emotional Health - Discusses mental and emotional health as a reflection of internal harmony, offering Arcturian techniques for treating anxiety, depression, and other mental and emotional disorders.

Chapter 18: Pain Treatment - Explores pain as a multidimensional communication mechanism, offering Arcturian techniques for relieving physical and emotional pain, including laying on of hands, energy acupuncture, and the use of crystals and essential oils.

Chapter 19: Women's Health - Discusses women's health as a reflection of the dynamic harmony between the physical body, emotions, mind, and spiritual energy, offering Arcturian practices for supporting women in different life phases.

Chapter 20: Child Health - Explores child health as a dynamic process of incarnation and learning, emphasizing the importance of creating high-frequency energy environments, fostering emotional bonds, and connecting with nature.

Chapter 21: The Importance of Mindful Eating - Discusses mindful eating as a way to reconnect with the essential energy of food, promoting presence, reverence, and the intentional choice of each element in the diet.

Chapter 22: Physical Exercises and Movement - Explores body movement as a natural expression of vital energy, highlighting the importance of conscious movement for maintaining energy flow, preventing blockages, and expanding body awareness.

Chapter 23: The Power of Restorative Sleep - Discusses restorative sleep as a multidimensional regeneration process, where the physical body, mind, and subtle bodies are restored and energetically realigned.

Chapter 24: The Healing of the Soul and Life Purpose - Explores the healing of the soul as a journey of reconnection with the purest essence of being, where the release of pain, the rescue of wisdom, and the alignment with life purpose converge.

Chapter 25: Integration with Conventional Medicine - Discusses the integration of Arcturian medicine and conventional medicine, highlighting the benefits of combining scientific rigor with vibrational and energetic depth.

Chapter 26: The Expansion of Consciousness and Planetary Healing - Explores the evolution of individual consciousness as an integral process that contributes to planetary healing, emphasizing the importance of self-realization, inner purification, and loving service to the collective.

Chapter 27: The Ethics of Arcturian Medicine in Practice - Discusses the ethical code that guides the practice of Arcturian medicine, emphasizing the sacredness of each being, the interconnection between subtle fields, and the importance of integrity, respect, and purity of intention.

Chapter 28: The Training of Arcturian Therapists - Explores the training process for Arcturian therapists, emphasizing the development of intuition, the practice of meditation and visualization, and the pursuit of self-knowledge.

Chapter 29: The Future of Arcturian Medicine - Discusses the future of Arcturian medicine, highlighting the integration of advanced technologies, the strengthening of intuition as a clinical tool, and the promotion of patient autonomy and planetary healing.

Prologue

As you delve into the words contained herein, you will not only encounter concepts and techniques of healing, but you will be gently led to question what it truly means to be healthy, balanced, and whole. There is something pulsing between each line, like an ancestral frequency that resonates with what is most intimate and authentic within you. It is as if the universe itself, in its silent wisdom, decided to deliver fragments of a lost knowledge, hidden under the dust of millennia, only for those willing to listen—and you are one of those chosen ones.

This is not an ordinary book about integrative medicine. It does not offer ready-made answers or simplistic formulas, but reveals a map, a hidden path that connects the physical body to the cosmic flows of energy and consciousness. It reminds us that healing is not just about eliminating symptoms, but about rescuing a sacred alliance between the inner self and the vibrant vastness that surrounds us. Each technique, each concept, and each practice described here is a key. And each key, in turn, opens portals that lead to truths far beyond the visible and the measurable.

Will you allow yourself to come into contact with knowledge that echoes from forgotten civilizations and cosmic intelligences that silently watch over the awakening of humanity? Will you have the courage to abandon the comfort of conventional explanations and dive into the brilliant abyss where science, spirituality, and mystery intertwine as parts of the same pulsating body? This is the invitation that this book extends to you—and not by chance.

The pages that follow hold secrets whispered through the ages. They speak of light technologies, subtle vibrational fields, and the invisible science of the soul. They reveal the indissoluble link between every emotion that crosses your chest and every cell that vibrates in your body. They show that your personal history, your beliefs, and even your silences are energetic codes imprinted on your subtle anatomy, shaping your physical, mental, and spiritual destiny. This book not only presents this knowledge—it activates it.

You will be guided by reflections and practices that transcend linear time and cultural boundaries, connecting ancestral Earth knowledge with the refined touch of a stellar wisdom that has long observed and awaited us. The Arcturian civilizations—whose name may seem distant or fabulous at first—are not just part of a cosmic mythology. They are guardians of an understanding so advanced that it manifests simultaneously as science and spirituality, as technology and reverence. By opening yourself to this knowledge, you do not only access information: you reconnect with parts of yourself that the modern world has taught you to silence.

With each chapter, with each suggested practice, you will notice something curious: the world around you will begin to show itself differently. Your subtle perceptions will sharpen, your emotions will reveal themselves as messengers, and your dreams will bring fragments of a cosmic memory that has never abandoned you. This book is not read only with the eyes, but with the expanded senses and the vibrational field of the soul. It is a mirror and a seed. It is a call and an initiation.

Be careful not to underestimate the impact of these words. They were written, compiled, and transmitted with a purpose: to awaken in you the desire to remember. To remember that health is flow. That balance is dance. And that living is, above all, remembering who you are before the layers and masks of everyday life. At this moment, as you hold this work in your hands, something has already been activated. An ancient frequency has recognized your current vibration and, silently, has begun the adjustment process.

Reading these pages is more than an intellectual choice. It is an energetic pact. Each word, each concept, each technique is an invitation for you to become the conscious co-creator of your own vibrational reality. You are not a passive spectator of your pains and cures. You are, and always have been, the alchemist of your own body, your mind, and your soul.

Therefore, allow yourself. Allow yourself to go beyond what you already know. Allow yourself to abandon comfortable skepticism and walk through this territory of mystery and light. This book is a map, a compass, and a master key. But the true portal can only be opened from within—by you. And it is already waiting.

May this reading be not only informative but transformative. May each page be a mirror where you finally see the bright and hidden truth of your own essence.

With respect and deep confidence in your journey,
Luiz Santos Editor

Chapter 1
Integrative Medicine

Integrative medicine is consolidated as a broad and innovative approach, capable of transforming the way health and disease are understood, diagnosed, and treated. Distancing itself from reductionist views that fragment the human being into isolated systems or into mere symptoms to be suppressed, this proposal is based on a systemic and integrative vision, where each dimension of existence—physical, emotional, mental, social, and spiritual—connects and influences each other. Health is no longer a condition restricted to the absence of detectable diseases in laboratory tests and becomes conceived as a dynamic state of balance, vitality, and harmony. In this context, body and mind intertwine in a continuous dance, where emotions and thoughts modulate biochemical and physiological processes, and physical conditions reverberate in the psychic universe. This integrative model does not deny or replace the advances of conventional medicine, but expands and complements them, incorporating traditional knowledge, self-care practices, and a deep appreciation for the uniqueness and autonomy of each patient.

Throughout human history, healing practices have always reflected the search for the restoration of this fundamental balance. Ancestral peoples, in different cultures, developed healing systems based on the connection with nature, the observation of life cycles, and the harmonization of internal and external forces. Traditional Chinese, Ayurvedic, and Indigenous medicines, for example, recognize the intrinsic relationship between body, mind, and spirit, and understand illness as the rupture of this essential harmony. With the advent of modern science, particularly from the 19th century onwards, there was a progressive fragmentation of this integrative view. The emphasis shifted to the detailed analysis of the parts, to the objectivity of quantifiable evidence, and to the direct combat of disease-causing agents. Although this approach has allowed extraordinary advances in the understanding of pathophysiological mechanisms and in the development of effective treatments, the subjective, symbolic, and existential dimension of human experience has, to a large extent, been disregarded. Integrative medicine emerges as a necessary counterpoint, rescuing this expanded view and promoting the reintegration of knowledge, practices, and perspectives that recognize the human being as a complex and interdependent unit.

Within this horizon, health care takes on a deeply humanized and participatory character, where the patient is no longer a passive recipient of interventions and becomes an active agent in the process of recovery and maintenance of their well-being. This paradigm shift involves the recognition of the biological, emotional, and spiritual individuality of each person, as well as their life trajectory, values, beliefs, support networks, and sociocultural context. Therapeutic interventions are co-constructed in a respectful and collaborative dialogue between health professionals and patients, integrating advanced diagnostic and treatment technologies with self-care practices, promotion of healthy lifestyles, and cultivation of meaningful connections with oneself, with others, and with the environment. Integrative medicine, therefore, does not represent a simple sum of techniques or disciplines, but a true paradigm shift, where the greater objective is to promote health in its fullest sense, encompassing physical well-being, emotional balance, mental clarity, social vitality, and spiritual connection—elements that are inseparable in the construction of a healthy and fulfilling life.

Historically, medicine has always incorporated elements of natural and spiritual healing, with healers and shamans who used herbs, rituals, and other practices to promote well-being. However, the development of scientific medicine, from the 19th century onwards, prioritized the study of the physical body and its diseases, relegating the subjective dimensions of human experience to a secondary role. Integrative medicine rescues this expanded view, seeking to integrate the knowledge of modern science with ancestral wisdom.

Health, from the perspective of integrative medicine, is not limited to the absence of disease, but encompasses well-being in all dimensions of being. A healthy individual is one who experiences vitality, emotional balance, mental clarity, and spiritual connection. Integrative medicine seeks to identify the root causes of imbalances, rather than just treating the symptoms. To do this, it uses a variety of tools, from laboratory and imaging tests to manual therapies, meditation, yoga, and nutritional counseling.

The interconnection between body, mind, and spirit is, undoubtedly, one of the central pillars that support the proposal of integrative medicine. In this expanded model of care, the human body is not seen as a fragmented machine, composed of isolated systems that function independently. On the contrary, each cell, tissue, and organ forms an intricate mosaic of interdependencies, where the harmonious functioning of one part reverberates throughout the organism and, likewise, imbalances in one specific area can echo throughout the system. This systemic understanding allows us to recognize that emotions and thoughts are not mere secondary products of brain activity, but active components in the field of health, directly influencing gene expression, immune regulation, hormonal balance, and physiology as a whole.

The connection between mind and body is especially evident when we consider the impact of chronic stress on physical health. Prolonged stress constantly activates the hypothalamic-pituitary-adrenal axis, triggering the excessive release of cortisol, a hormone that, in high doses and for prolonged periods, promotes a series of harmful changes. The immune system weakens, making the body more vulnerable to infections and chronic inflammatory processes. The walls of blood vessels suffer from increased blood pressure, and cardiovascular risk increases. The digestive tract, in turn, responds with functional disorders, such as gastritis, irritable bowel syndrome, and gastroesophageal reflux. Thus, persistent feelings of anxiety, anguish, and emotional overload leave concrete marks on the structure and functioning of the body, demonstrating how emotions shape physiology in real time.

This flow of influences, however, is not unidirectional. Physical state also exerts powerful influence over the mind and emotions. A body that is adequately nourished, in regular movement, and with restorative sleep cycles, provides the biological substrate necessary for emotional stability and mental clarity. The neurotransmitters responsible for mood regulation, such as serotonin, dopamine, and GABA, depend directly on the availability of essential nutrients, such as tryptophan, magnesium, omega-3, and B-complex vitamins. Likewise, the balance of the intestinal microbiome, composed of trillions of microorganisms that inhabit the digestive tract, is now recognized as a determining factor for mental health. The bidirectional communication between the intestine and the brain, mediated by the vagus nerve and bacterial metabolites, integrates the physical and psychic dimensions in a sophisticated way, reaffirming the indivisibility of the human being.

In this context, spirituality emerges as an equally relevant dimension for promoting health and resilience. Far from being understood exclusively as adherence to a formal religion, spirituality is recognized as the search for meaning, purpose, and connection with something greater—whether this force is understood as nature, the cosmos, humanity, or divinity. Contemporary scientific studies have shown that people who cultivate spiritual practices or have a strong sense of purpose have lower levels of systemic inflammation, greater resistance to stress, and better quality of life. This connection with the transcendent provides an inner foundation capable of sustaining the individual in the face of adversity, functioning as an anchor of emotional stability and a source of motivation for self-care and the maintenance of health.

By recognizing that each person is unique in their physical, emotional, and spiritual constitution, integrative medicine emphasizes the importance of personalizing treatments. This personalization transcends the simple choice of medications or therapeutic techniques, encompassing a careful look at the patient's life history, their beliefs, values, traumas, achievements, family environment, support network, and sociocultural context. Each individual carries with them a unique narrative, where health and illness intertwine with lived experiences and with the meanings attributed to each of them. In this sense, the therapeutic plan is constructed as a delicate craft, where each piece is shaped in dialogue between the health professional and the patient, respecting the rhythm, preferences, and limits of each person.

In this partnership relationship, the patient is invited to take an active role in their own healing process. This protagonism does not mean simply following prescriptions and guidelines, but developing autonomy to make informed decisions about their health, understand the signals that their body emits, and identify the factors that promote or compromise their well-being. This empowerment is cultivated through health education, attentive listening, and the strengthening of mutual trust between professional and patient, allowing each person to recognize themselves as an agent of their own vitality and balance.

Prevention and health promotion occupy a central place within integrative medicine, expanding the focus beyond the treatment of already established diseases. Primary prevention, for example, includes the adoption of daily habits that strengthen vitality and reduce the risks of illness. Among these habits, a balanced diet plays a fundamental role. A diet rich in natural and minimally processed foods is recommended, with an emphasis on vegetables, fruits, nuts, legumes, seeds, and fish rich in omega-3. The preparation of meals can be a therapeutic act in itself, especially when carried out consciously and connected to the present moment.

Regular physical activity complements this integrative care, adapted to the preferences and conditions of each person. From walks in nature to practices like yoga and tai chi, each movement contributes to the maintenance of flexibility, strength, circulation, and emotional balance.

Restorative sleep is another non-negotiable pillar. Creating a nightly ritual of deceleration, including reducing light and electronic stimuli, practicing deep breathing, and using relaxing infusions, such as chamomile or lemon balm tea, can help in the transition to deep and restorative sleep.

Stress management, in turn, involves the cultivation of relaxation and self-knowledge practices. Techniques such as meditation, conscious breathing, and journaling help to identify and process emotions, preventing the accumulation of tensions that can somatize into physical symptoms.

Health promotion goes beyond the individual sphere and reaches the community dimension. Belonging to support networks—family, social, or spiritual—strengthens resilience and nourishes the sense of connection, essential for well-being.

Thus, integrative medicine proposes a return to the essential: caring for the body, nurturing the mind, and feeding the spirit, recognizing in each daily choice an opportunity to reaffirm the commitment to life in its fullness.

In this way, integrative medicine reaffirms that health is not a stagnant state or a final destination, but a continuous process of construction and reconnection with oneself and with the world. By bringing together science and tradition, technology and listening, objectivity and subjectivity, this approach invites each person to assume the role of guardian of their own vitality, recognizing that genuine care arises from respect for one's own uniqueness and the invisible web that connects us to everything that exists. In this movement of re-encountering the essential, health ceases to be just the absence of pain or disease and becomes an expression of a conscious, integrated, and meaningful life.

Chapter 2
The Arcturian Civilization and Its Wisdom

The Arcturian civilization, originating from the star system of Arcturus, represents one of the most evolved and sophisticated cultures in the galaxy, both technologically and spiritually, presenting a model of existence based on absolute harmony between science, consciousness, and universal connection. Endowed with a wisdom that transcends the linear and fragmented knowledge of human civilizations, the Arcturians have developed a system of understanding reality where health, well-being, and spiritual evolution are inextricably intertwined. In their vast evolutionary journey, spanning millions of years, this civilization has built a society founded on full cooperation, the recognition of the sacredness of all life, and the conscious use of technologies that operate in tune with universal energy flows. This broad and integrated perspective allows the Arcturians to understand existence not only as a sequence of physical and temporal events, but as a continuous manifestation of vibrational frequencies, where matter, energy, and consciousness form a dynamic and interconnected web, reflecting the balance or dissonance of each being and each collective in relation to the cosmos.

This holistic view has profoundly shaped the way Arcturians understand health and healing, transforming the concept of medicine into something much more comprehensive than the simple elimination of symptoms or the fight against pathogens. For them, every manifestation of imbalance in the physical body is preceded and accompanied by disharmonies in the subtle levels of existence — emotional, mental, and spiritual fields that make up the energetic matrix of each individual. Illness, therefore, is interpreted as a rupture of the harmonious flow between the being and the universal energies that sustain it, and the healing process is much more than a mechanical correction: it is a vibrational reintegration, where the restoration of physical health is inseparable from the harmonization of emotions, the purification of limiting mental patterns, and the reactivation of conscious connection with the cosmic source. This understanding allows Arcturian medicine to be deeply preventive, acting in the preservation of internal harmony and in the maintenance of the continuous flow of vital energy before any disharmony crystallizes into physical symptoms.

The technology developed by the Arcturians reflects this deep integration between science and spirituality, incorporating healing devices that operate on quantum and subtle levels, capable of reading, interpreting, and modulating the energy fields of living beings. Their tools use specific patterns of light, sound, and sacred geometry to reorganize misaligned frequencies, dissolve energy blockages, and stimulate cell regeneration through precise and non-invasive vibrational processes. However, these advanced technologies are always applied in conjunction with practices of consciousness expansion, self-knowledge, and spiritual alignment, recognizing that true healing is inseparable from the awakening of consciousness and the reintegration of the individual into their greater purpose within the cosmic web of existence. By combining these elements — ancestral wisdom, quantum technologies, and a deeply integrative spiritual philosophy — the Arcturian civilization offers humanity not only healing techniques, but a new understanding of health as an expression of inner harmony and conscious connection with the whole, inaugurating a paradigm in which science, spirituality, and medicine converge to promote the integral evolution of the being.

Originating from a planet orbiting the star Arcturus, the Arcturians have developed, over countless eras, a society that reflects the pinnacle of conscious cooperation, where each being recognizes its unique importance within the living fabric of the collective, without ever losing awareness of its sacred individuality. In this social ecosystem, harmony is not imposed by rigid rules or authoritarian hierarchies, but emerges naturally from the deep understanding that the well-being of a single being reverberates throughout the social and energetic web that unites civilization as a single, vibrant organism. This vision rooted in the interdependence between all beings translates into daily practices where respect for all life — from microscopic organisms to beings of greater complexity and consciousness — is a natural expression of their own spiritual understanding. Among them, the concept of separation between science and spirituality is nonexistent, because for the Arcturians, exploring the mechanisms of matter and energy is just another way of understanding the emanations of the Primordial Source itself.

Arcturian technology is a direct reflection of this fusion between technical knowledge and spiritual wisdom. Mastering the manipulation of energy and light in its multiple frequencies, the Arcturians have developed ships capable of traveling not only through three-dimensional space, but also of penetrating the vibrational layers that connect different dimensional realities. Their vehicles traverse interdimensional portals and timelines with fluidity, using energy containment fields and frequency modulation that render mechanical propulsion obsolete. These same technologies of light and energy manipulation are applied in their medicine, architecture, and even telepathic communication, which is the primary means of interaction among members of this civilization.

Arcturian communication, based essentially on advanced telepathy, goes beyond the simple transmission of words or concepts. It involves the direct sharing of vibrational information packets, in which thoughts, emotions, images, and even complete memories are exchanged instantly, creating a form of dialogue where there is no room for misunderstandings or concealment of truth. This absolute transparency is the foundation of their culture, where truth is not an external imposition, but a natural expression of the vibrational integrity of each being.

Spirituality, within the Arcturian civilization, occupies a central and integrating position. Unlike human traditions, where the spiritual is often seen as something separate from everyday life, for the Arcturians, the evolution of consciousness is the very backbone of their existence. Every technological advancement, every healing practice, and every collective decision is guided by a relentless pursuit of expanded perception and the integration of new layers of cosmic truth. Arcturian philosophy emphasizes that evolution is not a straight line towards some point of arrival, but an ascending spiral, where each cycle of learning reveals new perspectives of the same infinite reality. The search for truth is, therefore, an act of loving surrender to the infinity of the cosmos, recognizing that all truth is provisional before the vastness of the unknown.

This intimate connection between spirituality and health manifests itself clearly in their healing practices, which go far beyond the mere removal of physical symptoms. The Arcturians master advanced energy healing techniques that involve reading, interpreting, and directly modulating the vital energy of each being. These practices are based on the premise that all illness is, before crystallizing in the physical body, a vibrational disharmony that runs through the emotional, mental, and spiritual fields. By directly manipulating these fields, the Arcturians are able to dissolve distorted patterns of energy before they become dense enough to manifest physical symptoms, making their medicine eminently preventive and deeply transformative.

For them, each being is a unique vibrational field, traversed by flows of vital energy that run through subtle channels — similar to the meridians described in traditional Chinese medicine — and converge in energy centers that we know as chakras. These energy centers, each with its specific frequency, function as points of intersection between the physical body and the subtle bodies, regulating the flow of information and energy between all levels of the being. When these flows are blocked or disturbed by crystallized emotional patterns, limiting beliefs, or unresolved traumas, internal harmony is broken and, eventually, the imbalance manifests as disease in the physical plane. Arcturian healing, therefore, consists of restoring the free flow of vital energy, removing blockages, and realigning each chakra so that it resonates again in harmony with the original vibrational matrix of the being.

Arcturian healing technology reflects this sophisticated understanding of energetic anatomy. Using devices that emit precise frequencies of light, sound, and sacred geometric patterns, the Arcturians are able to interact directly with the subtle fields, dissolving energetic congestions and reconfiguring the vibrational structures that support physical and spiritual health. These devices operate by resonance, identifying misaligned frequencies and emitting corrective pulses that restore the original balance, as if they were instruments tuning a vibrational orchestra. The same principles are applied in healing chambers, specially prepared environments where harmonic fields of light and sound create a space of high vibrational coherence, allowing for cell regeneration and energetic rebalancing in an accelerated and non-invasive way.

In addition to these technologies, the Arcturians also use their telepathic and telekinetic abilities in the diagnosis and treatment of diseases. Through telepathy, they can directly access the energy records of a being, reading their vibrational history and identifying the points of rupture and imbalance. Telekinesis, applied in a subtle and precise way, allows them to directly manipulate internal energy flows, removing blockages and redirecting vital energy as needed. These practices, however, are never performed invasively or unilaterally; they always occur in conscious collaboration with the being in the healing process, respecting their energetic sovereignty and free will.

Arcturian philosophy constantly reminds us that true healing is not an isolated event, but a continuous process of transforming consciousness. The liberation of negative patterns of thought and behavior, the dissolution of limiting beliefs, and the reconnection with the divine essence are inseparable elements of the restoration of integral health. Each act of healing is, ultimately, an act of remembrance — a recollection of who one is beyond the masks and layers accumulated throughout existence. Thus, Arcturian wisdom offers not only techniques and technologies, but a true path to integral healing, where body, mind, emotion, and spirit intertwine in a harmonious dance of self-recognition and awakening.

Integrating this ancient wisdom into human clinical practice does not mean rejecting the advances of conventional medicine, but rather expanding its boundaries. By recognizing the human being as a complex vibrational field, in constant dialogue with the cosmos, Arcturian medicine invites us to see health as a direct reflection of the harmony between the individual and the universal flow. This integration between terrestrial science and Arcturian wisdom has the potential to usher in a new therapeutic era, where advanced technologies and spiritual practices converge to promote healing on all levels, transforming not only medicine, but the very understanding of life and existence.

In this vast horizon of possibilities, Arcturian wisdom invites us to remember that true evolution lies not only in the accumulation of technical knowledge or in the mastery of external forces, but in the ability to align our personal vibrational field with the pulsating rhythm of the cosmos, restoring the natural flow between the being and the primordial source of all existence. By understanding that each symptom is a language of the spirit and each healing, an expansion of consciousness, we take the first steps to transform medicine — and the human journey itself — into a path of return to essential unity, where science and spirituality are not opposed, but intertwine as complementary expressions of the same infinite truth.

Chapter 3
Energy and Healing

Energy, understood as the essential substrate that permeates all of creation, establishes the basis for an expanded and integrative vision of health and healing, uniting ancestral traditions, discoveries of modern physics, and cosmic wisdoms that transcend human experience. Every being, every organism, and every structure existing in the material universe is, in its essence, a specific configuration of energy vibrating at a certain frequency, continuously interacting with the subtle fields that form the invisible fabric of reality. In the context of the human body, this energy manifests itself on different levels — from the bioelectrical flow that runs through the nervous and cellular systems, to the more subtle energy fields, such as the aura and the vibrational vortices known as chakras. Health, therefore, emerges as a direct reflection of energetic harmony, of the unimpeded and balanced flow of this vital force, which nourishes organs, cells, and systems, and at the same time interacts with emotions, thoughts, and states of consciousness, composing an inseparable dynamic between body, mind, and spirit.

Integrative medicine, by recognizing energy as the foundation of life and health, reintroduces into clinical practice a wisdom that has been present in numerous ancestral traditions, from the traditional medicines of India and China, to the shamanic healing systems of various indigenous peoples. All these traditions converge in the understanding that energetic balance is essential for the maintenance of health and that energetic disturbances precede, accompany, or even trigger physical and emotional symptoms. In the human system, the chakras function as regulating centers that process and distribute vital energy to the various organs and tissues, while the meridians form channels of energetic circulation that interconnect the different parts of the organism, creating an invisible network of communication and integration. Any blockage, deficiency, or excess of energy in these systems can be reflected in physical discomfort, emotional imbalance, or mental confusion, requiring interventions that restore free circulation and vibrational harmony.

The Arcturians, with their advanced understanding of energy as the primordial essence of all creation, further expand this vision by integrating science and spirituality into a single field of knowledge. For this cosmic civilization, vital energy is not only the foundation of individual health, but also the vibrational matrix that connects each being to the universal flow of existence. In their energetic medicine, each therapeutic process aims not only at restoring the internal flow of energy, but at reintegrating the being with the larger cosmic field, reestablishing the vibrational coherence between the individual and the universe. Techniques such as direct manipulation of light fields, the use of sacred geometries, and the application of specific sound frequencies are used to dissolve patterns of imbalance, stimulate cellular regeneration processes, and awaken expanded states of consciousness. By combining high-precision vibrational technology with a deep spiritual wisdom, the Arcturians offer humanity not only new therapeutic tools, but also a renewed vision of health as a state of deep vibrational alignment, where body, mind, spirit, and cosmos intertwine in a harmonious dance of light and energy.

The human body reveals itself as an energy system of intricate complexity, where each physical element finds its subtle correspondence in flows of energy that run through and sustain the totality of the organism. In this vibrational architecture, the energy centers, known as chakras, fulfill an essential function, acting as vortices that capture, process, and distribute vital energy to each organ, tissue, and body system. These chakras, arranged along the spine in an ascending sequence that goes from the base of the body to the top of the head, form a true energetic backbone, an invisible bridge between the physical and the subtle, between dense matter and the more ethereal layers of being.

Interconnecting these vibrational centers is a web of energy channels known in various traditions as meridians. These channels act as conductors that ensure the free circulation of vital energy throughout the body, creating a continuous network of communication between different parts of the body and allowing the subtle signals of vitality, balance, or imbalance to spread instantaneously through this integrated system. In harmony, these flows guarantee vitality, mental clarity, and emotional stability, sustaining the overall well-being of the human being. When this harmony is broken, whether by blockages, excesses, or energy deficiencies, the physical body, emotions, and even the mind begin to manifest signs of this imbalance, pointing to the need to reestablish the free and balanced flow of energy.

Vital energy, this essential breath that animates matter and sustains life in its multiple manifestations, is recognized by different traditions with different, but complementary, names. In the ancient Indian tradition, it is called prana, the cosmic force that permeates everything and nourishes every cell, every thought, every heartbeat. In Chinese medicine, it is known as chi, the subtle breath that circulates through the meridians and balances yin and yang, the complementary principles of existence. Whether as prana or chi, this primordial energy is absorbed from various natural sources, in a continuous process of exchange and nutrition. The air we breathe is impregnated with this subtle force, as well as the food we eat, especially those that are fresh, alive, and cultivated with respect for nature. Sunlight, in its full radiance, is also a direct channel of prana, nourishing not only the skin, but also the subtler layers of being, directly replenishing the energy fields that surround the physical body.

The constant and balanced flow of this energy through the chakras and meridians is what guarantees vitality and integral health. Each chakra, by receiving and radiating energy, feeds the corresponding organs and tissues, while the meridians function as vibrational rivers that distribute this vital force throughout the body. This delicate balance is dynamic, subject to internal and external influences, responding to emotional states, thoughts, the quality of the environments frequented, and lifestyle habits. When this flow is interrupted, obstructed, or diverted — whether by accumulated emotional tensions, physical trauma, or limiting mental patterns — the first signs of discomfort and disharmony appear. Disease, therefore, is rarely an isolated phenomenon; it arises as the final expression of an energetic imbalance that often began long before it became visible in the physical body.

Emotions, in turn, exert a profound influence on this energy field. Chronic stress, a phenomenon so present in modern life, has the power to constrict energy flows, stiffen meridians, and disturb the natural rotation of the chakras. This energetic compression directly affects the nervous system, hormonal and immune systems, paving the way for symptoms such as persistent fatigue, insomnia, recurrent headaches, and digestive disorders. Likewise, intense negative emotions — such as anger, fear, or deep sadness — not only affect the psyche, but also leave their dense impressions on the energy fields, creating areas of blockage and stagnation that, over time, can manifest as chronic muscle tension, unexplained pain, or even organic pathologies.

The mind, in its incessant dance of thoughts and beliefs, is another determining agent for vibrational health. Recurring thoughts of self-criticism, limiting beliefs about one's own worth or about the nature of reality create thought-forms that settle in the subtle fields as crystallized patterns. These patterns, in turn, affect the free flow of vital energy, altering the vibrational frequency of the being and predisposing it to imbalances both emotional and physical. Mental health, therefore, is inseparable from energetic health, both being faces of the same indivisible reality.

Within this panorama, the Arcturians offer an expanded and deeply sophisticated perspective on the nature of energy and its therapeutic applications. Understanding energy as the fundamental vibrational fabric that unites the entire cosmos, they see healing as a process of restoring the natural frequency of each being, returning it to its original resonance of harmony and coherence. Their advanced energy healing techniques combine precision vibrational science with a deep spiritual understanding of the nature of being. By working directly with vital energy, the Arcturians dissolve blockages, restore the fluidity of the chakras and meridians, and promote an integral realignment of the energy field, so that the body, mind, and soul pulse in unison again.

The basis of Arcturian energy healing lies in conscious intention and creative visualization, tools that, for them, are as concrete as any physical procedure. The Arcturian therapist begins each healing process by focusing their consciousness on a precise intention of healing, shaping the vibrational field around the patient with this clear purpose. Visualization comes as an essential complement, allowing mental images of harmony, light, and regeneration to be projected directly onto the energy fields in imbalance. These vibrational images are not mere subjective creations, but energetic molds that reorganize internal flows, as if each image were an activation key for the healing processes.

In some situations, the Arcturians use their own hands to channel energy directly to specific areas of the body or the auric field, acting as conscious conductors of cosmic energy. In other cases, they resort to sophisticated technological devices, capable of emitting specific frequencies of light and sound adapted to different patterns of imbalance. These devices function as vibrational tuning instruments, adjusting each chakra, each meridian, and each cell to its ideal frequency. Regardless of the technique applied, the central objective of Arcturian medicine is always the same: to awaken in the patient their innate capacity for self-healing, activating cellular regeneration mechanisms, strengthening natural immunity, and restoring the full connection between the being and its purest vibrational essence.

Healing, for the Arcturians, is not an external act imposed on the patient, but a collaborative process of remembering and restoring the original harmony. By restoring the flow of vital energy, dissolving emotional blockages, and reconfiguring limiting mental patterns, the human being is led back to their natural state of integral health — a state of alignment where body, mind, and spirit dance together in the same vibrational rhythm that echoes, in perfect resonance, with the very music of the cosmos.

Thus, energy reveals itself not only as an abstract concept or an invisible force, but as the primordial foundation of all experience of healing, self-knowledge, and evolution. Each restored energy flow is more than a physical adjustment: it is a vibrational reminder of the divine essence that inhabits each being, a subtle reconfiguration that allows body, mind, and spirit to express their unique melody in the infinite concert of existence. In this field of infinite possibilities, where science, spirituality, and consciousness intertwine, healing becomes a path of return to the natural state of harmony, where the human being not only exists, but vibrates in full harmony with the pulsating heart of the universe.

Chapter 4
The Chakras and Health

The chakras constitute a sophisticated energy system that transcends the simple notion of static energy centers, being understood as dynamic vortices in constant interaction with the physical body, mind, emotions, and spiritual fields that make up the totality of the human being. Each chakra operates as a point of convergence and distribution of vital energy, absorbing, processing, and radiating frequencies that reflect and influence the state of health and emotional and spiritual balance. In their primary function, the chakras act as bridges between the physical dimension and the subtle spheres of consciousness, connecting the organism to cosmic forces and telluric energies that flow from the planetary matrix itself. This continuous interconnection ensures not only organic functioning but also the expression of emotions, mental clarity, intuitive awakening, and connection with higher purposes, evidencing health as an expression of harmony between the material, psychic, and spiritual levels of existence.

The harmony and vitality of each chakra are shaped by personal experiences, emotional patterns, beliefs, and life habits, these energy centers being highly sensitive to the environment, relationships, and internal processes of each individual. When a chakra functions in balance, its rotation is fluid and its ability to capture and distribute vital energy is reflected in physical health, emotional stability, and mental clarity. However, blockages, overloads, or energy deficiencies in these centers can generate disturbances in different areas of life, triggering specific physical symptoms and promoting repetitive emotional patterns that reflect internal disharmony. A blocked heart chakra, for example, can manifest both in respiratory or cardiac difficulties and in difficulties in establishing genuine emotional bonds, while the imbalance of the throat chakra can impair both creative expression and thyroid health, illustrating the profound interdependence between the physical, emotional, and energetic bodies.

From the Arcturian perspective, chakras are seen not only as individual energy centers but as points of connection between the being and the vast cosmic network of intelligence and energy that permeates the entire universe. Each chakra is a vibrational portal that connects individual consciousness to planetary and galactic energy matrices, allowing the constant exchange of information and frequencies between the human microcosm and the universal macrocosm. The Arcturians, masters in reading and manipulating these subtle energies, use advanced technologies to scan, diagnose, and restore the harmonious functioning of the chakras, employing devices that emit coherent light and specific sound frequencies, capable of dissolving blockages, reorganizing energy flows, and recalibrating the vibration of the affected centers. This approach, associated with the development of self-awareness and spiritual expansion, allows not only the reestablishment of physical health but also the realignment of the individual with their higher essence and their evolutionary purpose, transforming healing into a process of cosmic reintegration, where body, soul, and universe begin to pulsate in harmonic resonance again.

The oriental tradition, in its millenary wisdom, recognizes and identifies seven main chakras, arranged in an ascending line along the spine, from the base to the top of the head. Each of these energy centers has a predominant color, a specific vibration, is related to an element of nature, corresponds to a gland and specific organs, and influences fundamental aspects of human experience, forming an energy map that reflects and governs physical, emotional, mental, and spiritual balance.

The first chakra, known as Muladhara or root chakra, is located at the base of the spine, near the coccyx. Its color is red, and its element is earth. It represents the foundation of existence, associated with survival, security, and connection with the Earth's telluric forces. This chakra is the basis of the survival instinct, regulating the individual's relationship with matter, the physical body, and the sense of belonging to the world. When balanced, Muladhara supports the feeling of basic security, material stability, and confidence to face life's challenges. When imbalanced, it manifests through irrational fears, constant insecurity, financial difficulties, and even problems in the bones, legs, and excretory system.

Ascending the spine, there is the second chakra, Svadhisthana, located in the pelvic region, below the navel. Associated with the color orange and the element water, it governs creativity, sexuality, and the natural flow of emotions. This energy center is responsible for pleasure, sensuality, and the ability to adapt to changes. When in harmony, Svadhisthana provides healthy pleasure, creative expression, and fluid and nourishing intimate relationships. However, when there are blockages, sexual repression, guilt, emotional coldness, or affective instability may arise, as well as problems in the reproductive organs and urinary system.

Just above, lies the third chakra, Manipura, located in the solar plexus, the region above the navel. Its color is vibrant yellow, and its element is fire. This is the center of personal power, willpower, and self-esteem. Manipura is the inner flame that drives self-confidence, the ability to make decisions, and the ability to manifest intentions in the material world. In balance, this chakra translates into inner strength, autonomy, and healthy self-esteem. On the other hand, when misaligned, it can generate low self-confidence, excessive passivity, or authoritarianism, as well as digestive disorders, ulcers, and problems in the liver and pancreas.

In the center of the chest, we find the fourth chakra, Anahata, the heart chakra. Its color is green, and its element is air. It is the balance point between the three lower chakras, linked to matter, and the three upper ones, linked to spirit. Anahata is the abode of unconditional love, compassion, and healing. When it is harmonized, it allows the full expression of feelings, the construction of healthy relationships, and the ability to forgive. Imbalances in this chakra can generate emotional blockages, difficulties in trusting and opening up, fear of rejection, and heart or respiratory problems.

Going up to the throat, we find the fifth chakra, Vishuddha, whose color is light blue and whose element is ether. It is the center of communication, authentic expression, and verbal creativity. Vishuddha governs the ability to express thoughts, emotions, and inner truth. In harmony, it allows expression to flow with clarity and creativity. When blocked, it can result in fear of speaking, difficulty in expressing oneself, or excessive defensive chatter, as well as problems in the thyroid, throat, and vocal cords.

Between the eyebrows, in the center of the forehead, lies the sixth chakra, Ajna, the third eye chakra. Its color is indigo, and its element is light. It is the center of intuition, inner wisdom, and seeing beyond appearances. Ajna regulates mental clarity, the ability to see the truth, and the connection with intuition. When in balance, it provides deep insights, discernment, and clarity. If blocked, it can cause mental confusion, excessive rationalism, or intuitive disconnection, as well as headaches, eye problems, and sleep disorders.

At the top of the head is the seventh chakra, Sahasrara, the crown chakra. Represented by the color violet or white, and associated with the element of pure consciousness, Sahasrara connects the individual to the divine and spiritual understanding. It is the point where the individual self meets the infinite, where limited perception dissolves into cosmic consciousness. In harmony, this chakra allows a sense of connection with the whole, inner peace, and deep understanding of life. When misaligned, it can generate a sense of existential emptiness, spiritual disconnection, or dogmatic fanaticism.

The balance of these centers is essential for maintaining physical, emotional, and mental health. When one or more chakras have excesses or deficiencies of energy, the symptoms manifest on multiple levels, from physical pain and specific illnesses to repetitive emotional patterns and existential crises. Muladhara imbalance can be reflected in chronic fears and financial insecurity. In Anahata, relationship problems and emotional isolation. And in Sahasrara, the lack of purpose and spiritual disconnection.

The harmonization of the chakras can be achieved through integrative practices that unite body, mind, and spirit. Guided meditation, for example, is a powerful tool. To practice it, sit comfortably in a quiet environment, close your eyes, and visualize each chakra as a sphere of vibrant light, from the base of the spine to the top of the head. Inhale deeply and, with each exhalation, imagine the light of these centers expanding and harmonizing. Repeat for 10 to 15 minutes.

The practice of yoga, with specific postures, also promotes energy alignment. Grounding postures, such as Mountain Pose (Tadasana), activate Muladhara, while chest-opening postures, such as Camel Pose (Ustrasana), stimulate Anahata. Conscious breathing (Pranayama), with a focus on the fluidity of vital energy, completes the process.

The use of crystals is another effective practice. To harmonize each chakra, choose corresponding stones: red jasper for Muladhara, carnelian for Svadhisthana, citrine for Manipura, green quartz for Anahata, aquamarine for Vishuddha, amethyst for Ajna, and clear quartz for Sahasrara. Place the crystal on the corresponding chakra during meditations or wear them as accessories close to the body.

Aromatherapy also offers vibrational support through essential oils. Put a drop of specific essential oil in your diffuser or dilute it in vegetable oil and gently apply it to the desired chakra. Use vetiver for the root chakra, sweet orange for the sacral, lemon for the solar plexus, rose for the heart, peppermint for the throat, lavender for the third eye, and frankincense for the crown.

In addition to traditional practices, Arcturian medicine adds a cosmic dimension to harmonization. Using telepathy and telekinesis, the Arcturians are able to scan the subtle fields and identify points of imbalance. By emitting coherent light beams and specific frequencies, they adjust the rotation and vibration of each chakra, promoting a deep realignment that restores the natural flow of energy and reconnection with higher consciousness.

These combined approaches allow the individual not only to restore their health but to reopen channels of communication with their essence and with the cosmic intelligence that permeates existence, realigning body, mind, and spirit in a harmonious dance with the universe.

In this way, the chakras cease to be just mystical concepts or symbolic elements of a distant tradition and become living maps, capable of revealing the energetic history of each being and guiding their process of healing and self-knowledge. When we recognize that every emotion, every choice, and every experience leaves its mark on this vibrational system, we understand that harmonizing the chakras is, above all, an act of reconnection with our own essence, an invitation to rescue the original fluidity of life and restore the dialogue between our physical, emotional, and spiritual aspects. By taking care of the chakras, we take care of the totality of the being, opening space for health, clarity, and purpose to flourish naturally, as an expression of a deep alignment between the human and the divine, between matter and light, between the internal pulse and the cosmic rhythm that surrounds and sustains us.

Chapter 5
The Connection with Nature

The connection between human beings and nature constitutes an ancestral, visceral, and inseparable relationship, where each natural element acts as a mirror and extension of the human essence itself. More than an external setting that serves as a backdrop for life, nature is the primordial matrix that nourishes, inspires, heals, and connects the individual to the living, pulsating network of the planet. Each leaf, river, mountain, and living being carries a unique energetic signature, a unique vibration that resonates with different aspects of the body and soul. The harmony between human beings and their natural environment is not just a matter of physical well-being or occasional leisure, but rather a vital necessity for the preservation of integral health, emotional balance, and the strengthening of spirituality. This deep bond, so often neglected by modern life, carries within it the potential to restore vital energy, calm the overloaded mind, and awaken the perception of belonging and interdependence with the whole, promoting a healing that transcends the body and reaches the very essence of existence.

The constant interaction with natural elements activates biochemical and energetic processes that sustain health and vitality. The simple act of walking barefoot on the earth allows the body to release accumulated electromagnetic charges and align itself with the Earth's energy field, a process known as grounding, which reduces inflammation, regulates biological rhythms, and strengthens the immune system. Exposure to sunlight, in addition to stimulating the synthesis of vitamin D, modulates the production of neurotransmitters such as serotonin and melatonin, directly influencing mood, sleep, and emotional stability. Contact with running water, whether in rivers, seas, or waterfalls, purifies not only the physical body but also the subtle fields, dissolving energetic tensions and promoting renewal and mental clarity. Each of these natural elements—earth, water, fire, and air—acts as a healing agent par excellence, adjusting the internal flows of energy, dissolving blockages, and facilitating organic and emotional self-regulation.

Beyond the physical and psychic benefits, the connection with nature opens portals of spiritual perception, rescuing an instinctive and intuitive wisdom that goes back to the first peoples of the Earth. The contemplation of natural cycles—the rising and setting of the sun, the phases of the moon, the blossoming and withering of the seasons—offers profound lessons about renewal, surrender, and impermanence. By observing these rhythms, human beings are invited to align their own internal cycles with the greater flows of life, recognizing themselves as part of a sacred web where every being, visible and invisible, plays an essential role in the balance of the whole. This perception, deeply rooted in indigenous cultures and equally understood by the Arcturians, reveals that true healing is not an isolated event that occurs only in the physical body, but a continuous process of reintegration of the individual into the living matrix of existence. In the Arcturian view, nature is both teacher and medicine, and the ability to consciously interact with its forces and intelligences is one of the foundations for full healing, the expansion of consciousness, and spiritual evolution.

Nature, in its generous and ancestral abundance, offers a true treasure trove of healing resources that span millennia and cultures, forming an invisible link between the earth and those who depend on it to sustain life and health. Among these natural gifts, medicinal plants occupy a prominent place. Used since time immemorial by indigenous peoples, shamans, healers, and medicine women around the world, they carry in their fibers, saps, and aromas properties capable of restoring the physical and energetic balance of the human body. Each plant, with its unique vibrational signature, possesses its own wisdom, a kind of living intelligence that acts in a subtle and powerful way, treating everything from simpler physical discomforts to deeper spiritual healing processes.

Preparing infusions, tinctures, and poultices from these plants is, in itself, an act of connection and reverence for the earth. The simple process of gathering fresh leaves at dawn, washing them with running water, and preparing an aromatic tea is already a healing ritual, where body, mind, and spirit intertwine in harmony. For a basic infusion, for example, simply boil 500ml of pure water, turn off the heat, and add a tablespoon of dried or fresh leaves of the chosen plant. Cover the container and let it steep for about 10 minutes, allowing the therapeutic properties to integrate into the water. Strain and drink, preferably in small sips and with full presence, feeling the warmth, aroma, and energy of the plant nourishing every cell of the body.

Crystals, in turn, are fragments of the planet's mineral memory, silent guardians of frequencies and information that echo since the formation of the earth's crust. Widely used in esoteric traditions and also revered in Arcturian medicine, crystals have the ability to act directly on the body's energy centers, the chakras, harmonizing them and re-establishing the healthy circulation of vital energy. Each crystal, with its color, composition, and vibrational structure, aligns with a specific need, functioning as a bridge between the subtle fields and the physical body.

To harmonize the chakras in a simple ritual, it is possible to lie down comfortably, preferably in a quiet space in contact with nature or with natural elements nearby, such as plants and water sources. Breathing should be slow and deep, leading the mind to a state of receptive relaxation. Then, specific crystals can be placed on each chakra: amethyst for the crown chakra, sodalite or lapis lazuli for the third eye, aquamarine for the throat, rose quartz for the heart, citrine for the solar plexus, carnelian for the sacral, and red jasper or obsidian for the root chakra. Remain lying down for about 15 to 20 minutes, allowing the energy of the crystals to act and rebalance the energy centers.

Water, this primordial and sacred element, is more than a chemical compound essential to life. It is the fluid memory of the earth, a vehicle for purification, renewal, and the constant flow of energy. In healing and reconnection rituals, whether in the context of Arcturian medicine or in the ancestral traditions of the Earth, water occupies a central place. Bathing in natural waters—whether in crystalline rivers, pulsating waterfalls, or saline seas—goes beyond physical cleansing; it is a symbolic and energetic act of releasing accumulated tensions, dissolving emotional blockages, and returning to the flow of life what no longer serves us.

At home, it is possible to recreate this sacred contact with water through therapeutic baths. To do this, fill a bathtub or basin with warm water and add a generous handful of coarse salt for energetic purification. The bath can be complemented with fresh or dried herbs, such as lavender, rosemary, or basil, and drops of essential oils according to the need of the moment. When entering the water, the body should be completely immersed, and breathing should be conducted consciously, inviting the water element to take away all tension, fear, or stagnant energy. Allow yourself to remain silent for a few minutes, listening only to the sound of your own breathing and the gentle contact of the water with your skin, creating a fluid and restorative meditation.

Pure air, this invisible vital breath that surrounds us, carries with it the memory of the wind, open fields, and ancestral forests. Breathing deeply in natural environments is not just a physiological act, but an invitation to nourish oneself with the living and vibrant energy that circulates among the trees, mountains, and valleys. Each conscious breath brings into the body not only oxygen but particles of life, of planetary memory, of cellular renewal. This simple act, when performed fully and presently, has the power to calm the mind, regulate emotions, and strengthen overall vitality.

Integrating this practice into daily life can be something simple, such as setting aside daily moments to walk in parks or green areas, breathing attentively, perceiving the texture of the air, the subtle scent of vegetation, and the dance of the elements in motion. Even in the most intense urban routines, opening a window in the morning, closing your eyes, and breathing in slowly, recognizing the air as a gift of life, is already a way of honoring this connection.

Sunlight, this inexhaustible source of energy and consciousness, is much more than just warmth and illumination. It is a code of cosmic information, carrying frequencies that activate biological, emotional, and spiritual processes. Responsible exposure to sunlight, especially in the early hours of the morning or the gentle moments of dusk, nourishes the body with vitamin D, regulates circadian cycles, and balances the production of hormones and neurotransmitters such as serotonin and melatonin, directly impacting mood, sleep, and general well-being.

The connection with nature, therefore, is not limited to sporadic moments of leisure or passive contemplation. It is an active and continuous practice of realignment with the greater intelligence of life, where each element—plants, crystals, water, air, and light—acts as a bridge and mirror between the self and the whole. With each barefoot step on the earth, each dip in living waters, each deep breath and sunbath, the physical body regenerates, the mind calms down, and the soul remembers its divine and earthly origin.

Arcturian medicine, in its cosmic wisdom, understands this integration as a fundamental part of full healing. For the Arcturians, true health arises from the balance between the physical body, the subtle fields, and the conscious relationship with the natural elements. They teach that each plant has a soul, each crystal is a guardian consciousness, each water source is a portal of renewal, and that learning to listen to these voices is to rediscover the path to inner balance. Thus, their healing practices include the use of specific medicinal plants for each energetic imbalance, carefully selected crystals to harmonize the subtle fields, and rituals of reconnection with the natural elements to restore the flow of vital energy.

Bringing this ancestral and cosmic wisdom into everyday life is an act of reconciliation with the essence of who we are. Walking in forests, cultivating a small garden, bathing in rivers and seas, observing the starry sky, planting and harvesting your own food—each simple gesture is a link that is remade in the great web of life. And so, by honoring nature in its multiple expressions, we also honor our own existence, rediscovering in the pulse of the earth the sacred mirror of our own soul.

In this reunion with living nature, human beings discover that their own healing is an act of reconnection with the earth, with the sky, and with the primordial flow that animates all forms of life. Every leaf that sways in the wind, every stone that rests silently, every dewdrop or ray of sunshine carries a silent invitation to remember that we are made of the same matter and the same light. By allowing ourselves to be silent and listen to this subtle language of nature, we rescue not only physical and emotional balance but also the ancestral memory that we are an inseparable part of a larger planetary organism, where every act of care for the world around us reverberates as deep care for ourselves.

Chapter 6
Arcturian Meditation and Visualization

Arcturian meditation and visualization form a field of practice that transcends the simple act of relaxing or directing the mind towards random images. It constitutes a refined spiritual technology, capable of realigning the human being with the universal flows of energy and cosmic intelligence. More than an isolated technique, these practices represent a vibrational portal for direct access to the higher spheres of Arcturian consciousness, a civilization that for millennia has mastered the art of harmonizing frequencies to promote healing, expansion of consciousness, and deep reprogramming of limiting internal patterns. Through the combination of clear intention, mental focus, and intuitive receptivity, Arcturian meditation allows the conscious mind to tune into subtle layers of guidance and healing, where flows of light and information are transmitted directly to the practitioner's energy field and vibrational core. This alignment not only dissolves emotional tensions and mental blocks, but also restructures distorted vibrational patterns, restoring coherence between the soul's purpose, the expression of the personality, and the overall health of the physical body.

When beginning an Arcturian practice, the first movement is the creation of a safe and elevated energetic field, a kind of inner temple where the mind, body, and spirit align with the frequency of pure light of Arcturian consciousness. This preparation involves purifying the subtle bodies, silencing the mental dialogue, and establishing a clear and loving intention of connection and healing. In this sacred inner space, the Arcturian golden light—a vibrational signature characteristic of this civilization—descends upon the practitioner, enveloping them in a field of protection and vibrational adjustment. This light acts as an energetic solvent, dissolving dense charges accumulated throughout life and adjusting the flow of vital energy in all force centers, harmonizing chakras, meridians, and auric layers. From this initial purification, the mind tunes into the Arcturian healing matrix, where geometric symbols, light languages, and subtle sound flows begin to manifest on the inner mental screen, transmitting encoded information directly to the spiritual DNA and the morphogenetic fields of the being.

Arcturian visualization, in this context, transcends the simple exercise of imagining scenes or landscapes and takes the form of a conscious mental technology, where each projected mental image is impregnated with precise vibrational intention and aligned with the universal principles of harmony and balance. Each mentally visualized symbol, color, or geometry acts as an access key, unlocking layers of information dormant in the energy field and reactivating the original potentials of the being, often obscured by traumas, limiting beliefs, and inherited emotional patterns. Consistent practice of these visualizations transforms the mind into a refined antenna, capable of capturing direct instructions from Arcturian consciousness, facilitating both self-healing and acting as a healing channel for others. Over time, the practitioner develops the ability to perceive, interpret, and direct subtle flows of Arcturian energy, becoming a conscious co-creator of their own vibrational reality and an active agent of their own spiritual evolution. By uniting meditation, visualization, and elevated intention, Arcturian practice reveals itself as a bridge between dimensions, a field of direct and continuous learning, where the human being and Arcturian consciousness co-create a new matrix of healing and expansion, aligned with planetary awakening and the integration of humanity into the cosmic family.

Arcturian meditation begins with the conscious creation of an inner sacred space, a kind of vibrational refuge where the mind, body, and spirit can align and rest in the serene and elevated frequency of Arcturian consciousness. This space is not a physical place, but a sensory field built with the power of intention, active imagination, and loving presence, becoming an inner portal for direct connection with the subtle spheres of this cosmic civilization. Creating this inner environment involves, first, finding a quiet physical place, a space where external silence serves as a mirror and support for the inner silence that will be cultivated. It can be a special corner of the house or even an outdoor space, as long as the practitioner feels safe, welcomed, and free from interference. In this environment, choosing a comfortable posture is essential, as the body needs to enter a state of receptive relaxation, where muscle tension and physical discomfort do not distract consciousness from the connection process.

Breathing then becomes the first key to accessing the sacred space. With deep inhalations and exhalations, the practitioner invites the body to abandon the accelerated pace of everyday life, allowing each cell to receive an infusion of serenity and presence. Conscious breathing, which deepens with each cycle, is the first signal to the energy field that the crossing is beginning, as if the inner atmosphere itself were being refined and adjusted, preparing the ground for the arrival of Arcturian light. In this state of quiet attention, the mind is gently led to the heart of the intention that guides this journey: to connect, learn, and receive healing directly from Arcturian frequencies. This clear intention is the vibrational anchor that allows the practitioner's personal field to tune in, like an antenna adjusting to the exact frequency of a specific cosmic signal.

With the intention established and the body in full receptivity, the next movement is to envelop the totality of the being in a white and golden light. This visualization is not only symbolic, but functions as an active vibrational tool, capable of reorganizing and purifying the subtle fields, dissolving accumulated energetic residues and adjusting the internal flow of vital energy. The white light carries within it primordial purity, a quality of crystalline clarity that dissipates dense and restorative patterns, while the golden light, with its Arcturian signature, imprints on the subtle bodies a frequency of harmonic adjustment and higher connection. This light, descending like a fine rain or a shimmering mist, envelops each layer of the being, penetrating from the skin to the deepest spiritual core, cleansing, adjusting, and preparing the vibrational ground for the conscious encounter with the Arcturian presence.

In this purified field, the practitioner then takes the next step: the direct invocation of the Arcturian presence. This invocation can be done through whispered words or just in thought, as long as the vibration of the intention is sincere and aligned with the heart. Words like "I invite the loving presence of the Arcturians to guide, heal, and teach me, in harmony with my Higher Self and the Divine Plan" can serve as a vibrational gateway, but each practitioner can find their own words, those that resonate with their essence and the nature of their moment of seeking. The power of the invocation lies not only in the words themselves, but in the quality of the presence that sustains them and the purity of the intention that animates them.

From this call, a subtle current of energy begins to flow, and it is in this flow that visualization transforms into a bridge between dimensions. The practitioner is invited to perceive this Arcturian energy not only as light, but as a living intelligence, capable of dialoguing directly with the body, mind, and soul. This energy penetrates the personal field, gently sliding through the subtle layers, reaching organs, tissues, and cells, where its frequency resonates like a silent song of healing and harmonization. Visualizing each part of the body being bathed and restored by this living light facilitates the reception of the healing flow and amplifies the vibrational adjustment. It is as if the Arcturian light found, within each cell, ancient and forgotten codes, awakening them and reactivating the original memory of health and harmony that exists in every being.

But Arcturian meditation is not limited to physical healing. It is also a profound tool for emotional release and mental restructuring. In this sacred space, the practitioner can visualize dense negative emotions, such as fear, guilt, or sadness, being gently dissolved and carried away by the stream of Arcturian light, like leaves being carried by a crystalline river. Likewise, limiting beliefs and mental patterns that create resistance to evolution can be surrendered to the golden light, which envelops them, resignifies them, and returns them to the practitioner as seeds of new understandings, more aligned with their higher essence.

This meditation also reveals itself as a portal to Arcturian wisdom, allowing information, guidance, and teachings to be transmitted directly to the practitioner's consciousness. As the mind becomes quieter and more receptive, subtle perceptions, insights, and even images or words that echo as telepathic messages from this advanced consciousness arise. This process of direct channeling is a skill that develops over time and with constant practice, making Arcturian meditation not just a moment of passive reception, but a living and dynamic exchange of information between dimensions.

To enhance this flow, Arcturian visualization can be directed towards specific purposes, such as creating detailed mental images of organs and cells being regenerated, or symbolic scenes representing the release of old emotions. Visualizing one's own energy field being recalibrated, or observing Arcturian geometric symbols descending in spirals of light and settling in the vibrational field, are practices that strengthen the connection and deepen the action of this spiritual technology.

In addition to self-healing, Arcturian visualization can also be directed to benefit others. By visualizing a person enveloped in the same golden light, being harmonized and healed, the practitioner acts as a channel, transmitting to the other's field the Arcturian frequency of healing and balance. This practice of distance healing, based on mental images and loving intention, always respects the free will of the other, operating only as a vibrational invitation that the person's soul can accept or not, according to their own evolutionary path.

Like any refined spiritual practice, Arcturian meditation and visualization require patience, discipline, and loving surrender to the process. Even a few minutes of daily practice are enough to strengthen the connection and refine the ability to perceive and interact with the subtle flows of this cosmic consciousness. Over time, the fusion of intention, meditation, and creative visualization becomes as natural as breathing, transforming into a state of expanded presence that permeates daily routine.

For those who want a basic structure to begin, the flow can follow these simple and effective steps:
1. Choose a quiet and silent place, sit or lie down comfortably.
2. Close your eyes and breathe deeply, relaxing the body and mind.
3. Visualize a white and golden light enveloping your entire being, purifying each layer of your field.
4. Invoke the Arcturian presence, with words or in thought, expressing your desire for connection and healing.
5. Feel or visualize the Arcturian energy flowing through your body, restoring harmony and balance.
6. Direct this light to specific areas that need healing or transformation.
7. Thank the Arcturian presence and end the practice slowly, maintaining the connection throughout the day.

Thus, Arcturian meditation and visualization, far from being just sporadic techniques, become a form of constant alignment between earthly consciousness and stellar wisdom.

In this continuous journey between worlds, Arcturian meditation and visualization reveal themselves not only as spiritual practices, but as a silent language capable of translating, in the body and soul, the impulses of a greater consciousness that gently reminds us who we are beyond the layers of time. Each encounter with this living light deepens the reconnection with the original code of our existence, dissolving the illusion of separation and awakening the memory that we are, also, part of this cosmic web of intelligence and love. By transforming the simple act of breathing and imagining into an intimate dialogue with the infinite, the practitioner not only receives healing or guidance, but rediscovers themselves as a living extension of Arcturian consciousness itself, a point of light in the process of remembering its original brilliance, co-creating a new vibrational reality for themselves and for the planet.

Chapter 7
Arcturian Energy Healing

Arcturian energy healing is an advanced practice of harmonization and vibrational restoration, based on the vast knowledge of an interdimensional civilization deeply connected to the universal laws that govern energy and consciousness. Unlike conventional therapeutic approaches, this modality understands the human being as a complex energetic system, whose frequencies and flows are directly influenced by emotions, thoughts, past experiences, and even ancestral and cosmic connections. Each individual is seen as a dynamic energy field, permeated by subtle layers that constantly interact with each other and with the environment. In this context, the Arcturians act as mentors and spiritual guides, offering healing technologies and sophisticated vibrational patterns that aim to restore the integral balance of the being, from the densest and physical levels to the subtle dimensions of the soul. This approach is not limited to the remediation of isolated symptoms, but seeks to reorganize the individual's energy matrix, promoting a harmonic resonance capable of sustaining continuous processes of self-transformation, expansion of consciousness, and spiritual alignment.

The essence of Arcturian healing lies in the understanding that vital energy—or the primordial cosmic force—is the fundamental matrix of all manifestation in the universe. Thus, diseases, emotional imbalances, and disharmonious mental patterns are direct reflections of interruptions or distortions in the flow of this original energy. By accessing Arcturian frequencies, the therapist acts as a conscious channel, establishing a vibrational bridge between the earthly sphere and the subtle high-frequency fields in which this evolved civilization dwells. This connection is not only through mental intention or creative visualization, but is sustained by a deep alignment of the heart, where the pure vibration of universal love resonates. It is through this loving attunement that the Arcturians transmit light codes and specific vibrational information, adjusted to the needs of each being. These codes, upon penetrating the subtle bodies, trigger processes of releasing cellular memories, dissolving blockages, and recalibrating the energy structure, allowing the vital energy to flow freely and harmoniously, reflecting on the physical, emotional, mental, and spiritual levels.

This therapeutic process is enhanced by specific techniques that increase the receptivity of the patient's energy field to Arcturian frequencies. Among these techniques are the conscious use of breathing as a tool for anchoring and amplifying the energy flow, the activation of sacred geometries that serve as vibrational frameworks to restructure fragmented fields, and the insertion of light codes directly into the main energy centers, the chakras. Each chakra, understood as a vortex of energy exchange between the human microcosm and the universal macrocosm, is carefully evaluated and harmonized to ensure the fluidity of vital energy. In addition, interdimensional telepathy allows the Arcturian therapist to perceive the most subtle nuances of the patient's energy field, capturing information about hidden patterns, soul contracts, or energetic records that directly influence the health and well-being of the being. By recognizing these deep layers of influence, Arcturian healing reveals itself not only as a practice of rebalancing, but as a path of profound self-knowledge, awakening the being to its true multidimensional essence and to its evolutionary purpose in the great cosmic fabric of existence.

Arcturian energy healing manifests as a practice that transcends simple energy manipulation, because in it every vibrational movement is conscious and guided by an intention deeply aligned with the original matrix of the being. Based on the ancestral and interdimensional wisdom of the Arcturians, this form of healing explores deep layers of the human energy field, where memories, records, impressions, and flows intertwine, creating the complex tapestry of experiences that shapes the life of each individual. The process begins with the anchoring of the therapist's consciousness, who, through internalization and connection with their own heart center, establishes the first vibrational link necessary to access Arcturian frequencies. This connection is not merely mental or imaginative, but a vibrational fusion in which the therapist's field expands to resonate with the more subtle fields of this civilization. Only through this pure attunement, free from personal agendas or egoic projections, can the therapist serve as a clean and integral channel for the healing energies that flow from the Arcturian plane.

The essence of this work consists of removing blockages, harmonizing the chakras, and restoring the fluidity of the energy field in order to allow the vital energy – this primary current that connects the being to the Source – to resume its natural flow, nourishing each layer of the being. The first step in this process is the initial reading of the energy field, performed through techniques of expanded sensory perception. The therapist, in a state of telepathic receptivity, "hears" the vibrations of the patient's field, capturing sounds, images, sensations, and even symbolic messages that reveal where the blockages are and what their origins are. This information emerges as subtle impressions or vibrational discharges that flow directly into the therapist's perceptual field, allowing them to understand not only where the energy has stagnated, but also which emotional, mental, or spiritual aspect needs to be welcomed, understood, and released.

After this initial reading, the therapist uses specific techniques to release the detected blockages. One of the fundamental tools is the conscious manipulation of energy through the focus and intentional direction of the vibrational flow. With the hands or only with the mind, the therapist guides the Arcturian energy to the points of stagnation, creating a continuous flow of light that envelops, dissolves, and transforms the dense particles accumulated over time. In many cases, these particles are residues of repressed emotions, obsessive thoughts, or crystallized traumas, which become true energetic knots in the individual's system.

Another fundamental aspect of the practice is the harmonization of the chakras, these vital centers that act as portals of exchange between the being and the cosmos. Each chakra is carefully evaluated, perceived in its tonality, frequency, and rhythm. A misaligned chakra may present opaque colors, irregular rotation, or even complete blockages, interrupting the free circulation of vital energy. To restore its harmony, the Arcturian therapist uses a combination of vibrational techniques, including the emission of specific tones, the activation of sacred geometries compatible with the original frequency of each center, and the insertion of Arcturian light codes, which act as recalibration keys, adjusting the vibration of the chakra to its ideal pattern.

This harmonization work does not occur in isolation, but within an integrated vision of the energy field as a whole. Each chakra, when realigned, directly influences the flow in the others, creating a vibrational cascade that restores the systemic harmony of the energy body. Therefore, the constant evaluation of the resonance between the chakras is essential, ensuring that no center is overloaded or left out of step with the others.

The manipulation of energy itself, known as a refined form of energetic telekinesis, is a skill developed by the Arcturian therapist throughout their journey of connection and practice. This telekinesis is not limited to the displacement of energy within the patient's body, but includes the ability to reshape flows, dissolve dense aggregates, and even insert informational packages directly into the subtle bodies. This insertion occurs when Arcturian light codes are anchored in the patient's energy field, acting as vibrational seeds that, over time, germinate into new perceptions, spontaneous unblockings, and natural realignments. These codes, in turn, are composed of geometric sequences of light, subtle sound patterns, and vibrational pulsations that resonate directly with the original matrix of the being.

In addition to telekinesis and telepathic perception, the use of high vibrational frequencies is a constant throughout the therapeutic process. These frequencies can be transmitted directly by the therapist's hands, channeled from the Arcturian field, or amplified through vibrational instruments such as crystal bowls, Tibetan bells, or even intuitively emitted vocal sounds. The purpose of these frequencies is to elevate the patient's vibrational field, creating a kind of "higher resonance field" in which dense blockages cannot be sustained, being naturally dissolved and transmuted. In some cases, specific crystals are used as vibrational anchors, potentiating the healing field and serving as stabilizing channels for the Arcturian frequencies.

The work with these crystals is done carefully and intentionally. Each crystal is previously cleaned, programmed, and tuned to the Arcturian frequencies before being positioned in the patient's energy field. Some crystals are placed directly on the chakras, while others are arranged around the body, forming geometric patterns that function as harmonization portals. The choice of crystal and its position is guided by the intuitive reading of the energy field, ensuring that each element acts in perfect synchrony with the specific needs of that being.

The removal of energy blockages, in turn, is one of the central pillars of this approach. These blockages can originate from a multitude of experiences and influences: unprocessed emotional traumas, self-sabotaging thought patterns, inherited limiting beliefs, or even energetic impressions of external origins, such as spiritual interferences or karmic records. Each blockage is treated as a crystallized expression of an unresolved story, which needs to be recognized, understood, and released. This release process, although often subtle, can manifest physically through thermal sensations, tremors, tears, or even spontaneous memories that emerge to be integrated and transcended.

The human energy field, known as the aura, is continuously evaluated and adjusted throughout the entire process. This outer layer of the being, which functions as a vibrational shield and as an interface of exchange between the internal microcosm and the universal macrocosm, is carefully cleaned, strengthened, and recalibrated to reflect the restored harmony in the internal levels. Any fissure, accumulation, or interference is identified and treated, ensuring that the energy field is whole and resonating at its highest and healthiest frequency.

Throughout the entire process, the pure intention and alignment of the therapist with the Arcturian consciousness are the foundation that supports each technique, each vibrational emission, each subtle adjustment. More than an executor of procedures, the therapist is a conscious co-creator of the sacred healing space, where patient and therapists are equally responsible for anchoring harmony and reconnecting with the primordial essence. Arcturian energy healing, therefore, is not just a technique, but a sacred dance between fields, consciousnesses, and frequencies, where each movement is a step on the path of return to the true multidimensional nature of the being.

In this flow where spiritual science and cosmic love intertwine, Arcturian energy healing reveals itself as a journey of reintegration of the soul to its original matrix, restoring in the being the living memory of its unbreakable connection with the All. Each vibrational emission, each geometry of light, and each subtle adjustment not only undoes blockages and dissolves densities, but opens internal doors for the being itself to reclaim its vibrational sovereignty, assuming the role of conscious guardian of its energy field and its evolution. In this healing space, the Arcturians do not position themselves as external saviors, but as loving mirrors that reflect the latent potential of each being to become their own healer, their own master, remembering that true healing is always a return: to the center, to the silence, and to the primordial song that resonates in the heart of existence.

Chapter 8
Using Crystals and Sacred Geometry

The use of crystals and sacred geometry within Arcturian medicine represents a sophisticated synthesis of spiritual science and vibrational technology, reflecting a deep understanding that all creation is structured by geometric patterns and specific frequencies. Crystals, by their very molecular nature, function as condensers and amplifiers of cosmic energy, capturing, storing, and retransmitting specific vibrations that interact directly with the human energy field and the subtle flows that permeate the physical, emotional, mental, and spiritual bodies. This interaction occurs because each crystal emits its own frequency, a result of its chemical composition, internal structure, and geological origin, making it a kind of natural antenna tuned to certain aspects of universal consciousness. When used consciously and intentionally, crystals become powerful tools for restoring harmony, dissolving energy blockages, and facilitating processes of healing and consciousness expansion, acting as catalysts for beneficial resonances and reorganizers of misaligned vibrational patterns.

Sacred geometry, in turn, is not just a set of symbolic forms, but a primordial cosmic language, whose geometric patterns mathematically express the underlying order that organizes matter and energy at all levels of creation. Present from cellular and molecular structures to the organization of galaxies, sacred geometry represents the vibrational map of manifestation, where each shape, angle, and proportion carries within it a specific energy code, capable of restoring the coherence of the vibrational field of individuals, environments, or even collective processes. When applied alongside crystals, sacred geometry potentiates and directs the healing properties of these natural elements, creating resonance circuits that amplify the effectiveness of energy harmonization. Crystal grids arranged in specific geometric patterns act as true multidimensional antennas, connecting physical space with higher frequencies, promoting lasting energetic stabilization, and serving as portals for receiving light codes and information from higher spheres of consciousness.

By integrating crystals and sacred geometry into Arcturian healing practices, the therapist or practitioner not only enhances the efficiency of the energetic intervention but also anchors subtle high-vibration frequencies in the physical plane, creating environments conducive to the deep realignment of the personal energy matrix. This integration, however, requires more than technical knowledge; it demands a refined attunement to the consciousness of crystals, an intuitive understanding of geometric relationships, and the ability to act as a conscious channel between dimensions. Each crystal selected resonates with a specific aspect of the individual's psyche and energy body, and each geometric form used in the process interacts directly with the subtle fields, activating or restoring interrupted flows. Thus, the alliance between crystals and sacred geometry not only complements other Arcturian healing techniques but also offers a profound path of reconnection with the original matrix of the soul, facilitating the release of limiting patterns, the activation of dormant potentials, and the construction of a new energetic structure capable of sustaining expanded states of consciousness and full vibrational health.

Each crystal used within Arcturian medicine carries unique healing properties and specific vibrations that resonate with different aspects of the human being, whether on a physical, emotional, mental, or spiritual level. These mineral beings, formed over geological eras, hold in their atomic structures the memory of the Earth and the cosmic forces that shaped them, becoming true guardians of vibrational wisdom. Rose quartz, for example, is one of the most well-known and revered crystals when it comes to emotional healing. Its frequency is gentle yet profound, radiating a compassionate energy that envelops the auric field like a gentle embrace, dissolving layers of accumulated pain and emotional scars. The mere presence of this crystal near the heart seems to soften tensions and reopen internal portals to acceptance, self-esteem, and unconditional love, not only in relation to others but mainly towards one's own essence.

Amethyst, in turn, carries a higher, almost ethereal vibration, capable of acting as a purifier of dense thoughts and emotions. With its violet color, which symbolizes spiritual transmutation, amethyst is widely used in meditative practices, helping to quiet the mind and amplify intuition. Its energy creates a subtle bridge between the earthly and spiritual planes, facilitating the reception of insights and the release of limiting mental patterns. More than just an amulet of serenity, amethyst is a vibrational portal that invites consciousness to expand beyond everyday illusions, connecting it with more subtle dimensions of the soul itself.

Meanwhile, black tourmaline, with its dense and opaque appearance, plays an essential role in protection and grounding. Unlike crystals that elevate the mind and spirit, black tourmaline anchors the being to the core of the Earth, creating a line of energetic support that allows deep healing processes to occur safely. Its dense frequency acts as a natural filter, absorbing and neutralizing dissonant energies that approach the auric field. More than just repelling unwanted external energies, it also helps to unveil and dissolve inner shadows, those hidden layers of fear and limiting beliefs that resonate with low-vibration energies. By acting as a shield and mirror, black tourmaline reveals what needs to be faced and transformed within oneself.

The selection of which crystal to use in each practice is always an act of attunement and intuitive listening. Although there are traditional properties associated with each stone, it is the silent dialogue between crystal and practitioner that reveals the true need of the moment. The same crystal can act in different ways in different contexts, as it responds not only to the expressed intention but also to the subtle layers that the soul silently manifests. Therefore, before each healing or harmonization session, it is essential to take a moment to silence the mind and allow the vibrational connection between therapist, crystal, and the recipient's energy field to establish itself naturally and fluidly.

The practical application of crystals in Arcturian medicine unfolds in various possibilities, each adapted to the purpose and nature of the necessary energetic intervention. In individual meditative practices, the simple act of holding a crystal in one's hands or placing it on a specific chakra is enough to establish a vibrational bridge between the personal field and the healing frequency of the crystal. This technique, although simple, requires full presence and a clear intention, as it is the fusion between consciousness and mineral that activates the full potential of healing.

Another widely used method is the placement of crystals on the body in energy harmonization sessions. In this case, each stone is strategically positioned on the chakras or on sensitive energy points, creating a resonance circuit that reorganizes interrupted flows and dissolves vibrational knots. Each crystal acts as an access key, unlocking internal portals and facilitating the release of emotional memories and ancestral patterns that are stored in cellular records.

In addition to direct application to the body, the creation of crystal grids represents one of the most sophisticated and potent techniques of Arcturian medicine. In these grids, specific combinations of crystals are arranged in precise geometric patterns, forming true energy circuits that radiate healing vibrations to the environment and to all who pass through. The energy of each crystal intertwines with the sacred geometry used, creating a cohesive field where the mineral force and the geometric code potentiate each other.

Another subtle, yet extremely effective resource is the preparation of crystal waters. By submerging specific crystals in pure water—always respecting which crystals can be used in direct contact with water—a vibrational infusion is created that transfers the healing properties of the stone to the water. This water can then be ingested or used to spray environments and auric fields, promoting a continuous and gentle vibrational purification.

Sacred geometry, intertwined with this work with crystals, manifests the very language of the cosmos. Patterns such as the Flower of Life, the Seed of Life, and Metatron's Cube are not mere symbols; they are vibrational maps that organize and sustain manifestation at all levels. Each line, each intersection, each proportion carries within it a specific frequency, capable of aligning personal and collective energy fields with the primordial cosmic order.

Visualizing and meditating with these symbols not only activates ancestral memories stored in the spiritual DNA but also reactivates dormant codes that hold the original blueprint of the soul. Within Arcturian medicine, this practice is not only contemplative but also active and intentional. By visualizing or tracing these patterns during healing practices, the therapist becomes a conscious co-creator, adjusting the vibrational matrix of space and being to the frequency of primordial harmony.

The creation of a crystal grid for protection is a clear example of this fusion between crystals and sacred geometry. This process begins with the careful selection of crystals whose frequency resonates with protection and strengthening of the auric field. Black tourmaline, onyx, and smoky quartz are common choices for their ability to create dense and effective vibrational shields. With the crystals selected, the appropriate geometric pattern is chosen, such as the Flower of Life, whose intersections spiral energy in multiple directions, or Metatron's Cube, which organizes space into perfect harmonic fields.

After the selection, each crystal must be cleansed and energized, removing remnants of previous energies. This purification can be done by exposing them to sunlight or moonlight, smudging them with sacred herbs, or using the sound of bells and crystal singing bowls. With the crystals prepared, the arrangement in the chosen geometric pattern begins, guided by both the external design and internal intuition. Finally, the grid is activated by consciously visualizing the energy flowing between the crystals, weaving lines of light that form a cohesive protective network.

This grid, once activated, should be positioned in strategic locations—in the bedroom, meditation room, or work environment—where its vibrational presence serves as a continuous shield and anchor point for high frequencies. Thus, the fusion between crystal and sacred geometry manifests not only as a protection tool but as a constant reminder that harmony and connection with cosmic order are natural states of being.

In the convergence of crystals and sacred geometry, a path of ancestral reconnection is revealed, where matter and light dialogue in silence, reestablishing bridges between the visible and the invisible. Each crystal, with its geological memory and unique vibration, becomes a guardian of internal portals, while each sacred form resonates as a master key, reactivating forgotten codes in the recesses of the soul. Together, they form a primordial language that speaks directly to the light body, reminding us that true healing is not an external intervention, but an invitation to return to the vibrational center where the essence and the Source recognize themselves as one. By intertwining these two fields of wisdom and power, the Arcturian practitioner not only harmonizes individual energy but also anchors on the earthly plane the very language of the cosmos, restoring in the here and now the perfect echo of the divine geometry that sustains all creation.

Chapter 9
Arcturian Aromatherapy

Arcturian aromatherapy manifests as an advanced practice of vibrational harmonization, where essential oils are understood not only as botanical extracts with therapeutic properties, but as carriers of specific frequencies tuned to the subtle fields of being. Each essential oil is seen as a concentrate of vibrational information from the plant of origin, capturing not only its chemical and physical properties, but also its primordial energetic essence, shaped by the interaction between the plant and the natural elements throughout its life cycle. Within this Arcturian perspective, essential oils act as olfactory light codes, capable of penetrating the most subtle energetic layers of the individual, promoting the recalibration of the vibrational field, unblocking energy flows, and restoring harmony between body, mind, and spirit. The aroma, then, ceases to be just a sensory experience and becomes a vibrational bridge that connects the human being to the wisdom of plants and, consequently, to the universal knowledge of the healing matrix present in nature and amplified by Arcturian spiritual technologies.

Each essential oil, in the Arcturian view, carries a unique vibrational signature that resonates with certain aspects of human consciousness and energy centers. Lavender, for example, carries the frequency of cosmic serenity, dissolving emotional tensions and restoring harmony between the subtle bodies. Lemon vibrates in tune with mental clarity and energetic purification, acting as an agent that disperses miasmas and accumulated densities in the auric field. Rose oil, in turn, radiates the frequency of universal love, promoting the healing of ancestral emotional wounds and restoring the connection with self-love and divine self-esteem. In Arcturian practice, the choice of an essential oil is not guided only by the physical or emotional symptoms presented, but by the vibrational reading of the individual's energy field, allowing the oil most compatible with the frequency and evolutionary moment of the being to be applied. This intuitive and conscious selection creates a field of resonance between therapist, patient, plant, and Arcturian energy, where each component acts as part of a larger flow of cosmic intelligence in action.

The application of essential oils in Arcturian aromatherapy expands beyond traditional practices, incorporating techniques of energetic tuning, creative visualization, and anchoring of higher frequencies. The simple act of inhaling an aroma becomes a process of conscious reception of vibrational information that awakens cellular memories of healing, releases stored traumas, and reactivates dormant light codes in the energetic DNA. In therapeutic sessions, the Arcturian therapist can combine the application of oils with the projection of sacred geometries in the patient's energy field, using the aroma as an anchoring vehicle for these vibrational forms. It is also common to use aromatic grids, where different oils are arranged in specific geometric patterns, creating fields of aromatic resonance that act in environmental harmonization, in the strengthening of sacred spaces, and in the amplification of healing intentions. This expanded view of aromatherapy, where fragrance is only the sensory manifestation of a broader cosmic frequency, transforms the relationship with essential oils into a direct dialogue with the intelligence of nature and with Arcturian consciousness, promoting not only the healing of symptoms, but the deep reconnection with the vibrational essence of being and with its evolutionary purpose within the cosmic web of creation.

Each essential oil, within the refined practice of Arcturian aromatherapy, manifests a unique vibrational signature, which interacts directly with different layers of consciousness and with the energy centers that sustain the integrity of being. Each essence carries with it the vibrational memory of the plant from which it was extracted, reflecting not only its chemical properties, but the deep interaction that that life form established with the elements of the Earth and with the cosmic cycles that shape planetary existence. In this context, lavender essential oil is recognized as a true vibrational balm, whose calming and relaxing frequency harmoniously intertwines with the subtle fields, dissolving accumulated tensions and restoring the natural flow of internal energies. Upon coming into contact with the auric field or being consciously inhaled, lavender acts as a violet mist of serenity, which travels through the invisible fibers of the mind and the energy body, dissolving anxieties, calming mental agitation, and facilitating the return to the inner axis of balance. Its action extends to the processes of sleep and psychic regeneration, assisting not only in inducing physical rest, but in opening dream portals where ancestral memories and higher insights can be accessed with clarity and safety.

Within this same vibrational web, lemon essential oil resonates like a ray of golden light that pierces the auric field with its purifying and invigorating energy. The presence of this citrusy and luminous aroma has the power to disperse energetic miasmas accumulated around the subtle body, dissolving fields of stagnation and releasing the vital energy that often remains trapped in dense pockets of repetitive thought or crystallized emotion. At the same time, its vibrational signature stimulates mental clarity and the reorganization of thought patterns, as if each molecule of the aroma were a renewing breath that sweeps away psychic dust and realigns the flow of ideas with the clear geometry of the higher mind. This oil, when integrated into daily practices, acts not only in strengthening the physical immune system, but also in reinforcing energetic immunity, creating a field of luminous vitality that repels dissonant external influences.

Rose essential oil, in turn, walks another path within Arcturian medicine. Its deep, sweet, and enveloping aroma carries in each drop the vibration of unconditional love and universal compassion. It acts directly on the most delicate layers of the emotional field, dissolving armor built up over painful experiences and softening invisible scars that remain stored in the folds of affective memory. Upon coming into contact with the heart's energy field, the rose whispers ancient memories of belonging and acceptance, reminding the soul of its natural capacity to love and be loved, to give and receive in free and constant flow. More than just a tool for emotional healing, rose oil rescues the soul's own original frequency in its purest expression, connecting each being to its capacity to radiate self-love, nurture authentic bonds, and dissolve relational patterns based on fear or lack.

The selection of an essential oil within the Arcturian practice, therefore, goes far beyond choosing a pleasant aroma or treating isolated symptoms. Each choice is a vibrational reading, an intuitive recognition of what that specific energy field needs at that moment in its evolutionary journey. Therefore, before any application, the Arcturian therapist or practitioner quiets the mind and tunes into the subtler layers of the individual's energy, allowing the resonance between essence and being to reveal which oil wishes to be the healing agent at that moment. This refined listening allows each drop applied to be not just a physical substance, but a coded vibrational message, capable of reorganizing patterns, releasing memories, and restoring essential harmony.

The application of essential oils in Arcturian practice unfolds in multiple possibilities. In its simplest and most direct form, they can be used in environmental diffusers, where their fragrance subtly spreads through the space, permeating the environment with their healing frequencies and creating a field of protection and harmony. Each breath in this environment becomes a conscious reception of the vibrational information of the oil, which integrates into the practitioner's field in a gentle and continuous way. This technique is especially used to prepare meditation rooms, therapeutic spaces, or even home environments, transforming them into true vibrational temples where body, mind, and soul can rest and regenerate.

Another form of application, equally powerful, is direct inhalation. By dropping a drop of essential oil on a handkerchief or personal inhaler, the practitioner allows the aromatic molecules to enter directly into the respiratory system and reach the limbic system, where memories, emotions, and ancestral patterns are processed and reorganized. This technique is particularly effective for dealing with acute emotional crises, episodes of anxiety, or respiratory blockages of energetic origin, where the aroma acts as a key to rapid and effective release.

Aromatic massages are another expression of this sacred integration between plant and human being. When diluted in high-purity vegetable oils, essential oils can be applied directly to the skin, allowing their frequencies to penetrate the physical and energetic layers simultaneously. Each movement of the massage becomes a conscious gesture of connection, where the skin, the aroma, and the intention of the touch form a healing circuit that harmonizes muscles, emotions, and vibrational patterns. The same principle applies to localized topical application, where small portions of diluted essential oil can be used to treat specific areas of the body or energy points that need special attention.

In more advanced cases, the ingestion of essential oils, always under the guidance of a qualified professional attuned to the Arcturian vision, can be used as a complementary tool. In these cases, the essence acts directly on the internal systems, reorganizing vibrational patterns from the physical center of being.

Synergies, carefully harmonized combinations of essential oils, represent another facet of this refined practice. A classic combination used in Arcturian medicine to promote deep relaxation and emotional balance is the union of lavender, chamomile, and marjoram. Together, these essences create a field of loving serenity that calms the mind and heart, preparing the vibrational field for meditative processes or for restorative rest. Likewise, the combination of lemon, eucalyptus, and rosemary creates a vibrationally invigorating synergy, which strengthens the immune system and clarifies mental flows, dissipating confusion and stagnation.

Regardless of the technique or combination chosen, pure intention and conscious connection with the essence of each oil are the foundation on which the entire Arcturian practice is based. Before each application, the practitioner is invited to enter a meditative state, silence the mind, and open the heart, allowing the connection with the vibrational essence of the oil to be established at its purest level. At the end of each application, the act of thanking the essence and the plant consciousness that sustains it is not just a spiritual formality, but a form of recognition and alignment with the network of intelligence that permeates all creation.

In this way, Arcturian aromatherapy reveals itself not only as a therapeutic technique, but as a journey of subtle and deep reconnection with the vibrational essence of being, where each aroma, each molecule, and each breath are portals to remember who we are and to realign our presence with the cosmic symphony of which we are a part.

In the invisible essence of each aroma pulses an ancestral history of connection between realms, where plant and human being meet as vibrational mirrors of the same expanding consciousness. In Arcturian practice, this subtle exchange transforms each inspiration into an act of remembrance, where fragrance becomes the messenger of a living wisdom that speaks directly to the soul, dissolving layers of forgetfulness and restoring the fluidity between mind, body, and spirit. By aligning plant memory with the vibrational geometry of being, Arcturian aromatherapy not only heals or relieves, but returns to the practitioner the awareness of their interdependence with the whole, reminding us that the perfume of plants is, in essence, the whisper of the Earth itself guiding each soul back to its original melody.

Chapter 10
Arcturian Breathing Techniques

Arcturian breathing techniques represent a refined synthesis between energetic science and cosmic wisdom, where the act of breathing transcends its biological function and becomes a vibrational key to accessing expanded states of consciousness, harmonizing internal energy flows, and reconnecting the human being to the universal web of energy and information. For the Arcturians, each respiratory cycle is an opportunity to recalibrate the energy structure, dissolve accumulated blockages, and restore the free circulation of vital energy through all the subtle bodies. The air that enters the airways is understood as a vehicle carrying encoded light particles, known as cosmic prana, which transport healing frequencies directly from the higher spheres to the individual energy field. This continuous flow of subtle energy, when directed with conscious intention and associated with specific visualizations, has the power to reprogram cells, rebalance energy centers, and harmonize misaligned vibrational patterns that impact physical, emotional, and mental health.

The Arcturian practice of conscious breathing is carefully adjusted to act as a communication channel between the individual and the higher spheres of light, allowing each breath to bring not only oxygen to the physical body but also vibrational information that nourishes the auric field and resonates with the light codes present in the energetic DNA. In this context, breathing ceases to be just an automatic act and becomes a sacred process, where each respiratory cycle is an opportunity to reset crystallized emotions, release memories of pain, and activate conscious presence in the here and now. By breathing consciously, the individual expands their capacity for subtle perception, becoming able to clearly identify the areas of the body or energy field where there is stagnation or vibrational fragmentation. This guided perception allows the breath to be directed as an active therapeutic tool, dissolving energetic congestion and reactivating the fluidity necessary for integral well-being. In this way, Arcturian breathing acts as a direct portal to self-listening, self-knowledge, and the alignment of the personality with the soul's higher purpose.

Within the Arcturian repertoire, some specific breathing techniques are widely used to promote cleansing, strengthening, and protection of the energy field. Cyclic breathing, for example, combines deep inhalation, conscious retention, and prolonged exhalation, creating an energetic pulsation that resonates with the cosmic heartbeat and facilitates synchronization between the cerebral hemispheres. This technique is particularly effective for releasing stored traumas, deconstructing repetitive thought patterns, and accessing deep meditative states, in which insights and higher guidance can be received clearly. Another widely practiced technique is the tube of light breathing, where the individual visualizes a beam of light that passes through their entire central axis, connecting heaven and earth, while conscious breathing activates the upward and downward flow of this healing light. This practice creates a natural energy shield, strengthens the connection with the Higher Self and with the Arcturian consciousness, and establishes a continuous resonance between the personal vibration and the harmonic frequencies of the universe. By integrating these breathing practices into the daily routine, the individual not only takes care of their physical and emotional health but also develops a deep sense of cosmic belonging, recognizing themselves as an active part of the universal web of light and regaining their energetic sovereignty as a conscious co-creator of their own reality.

Conscious breathing, the essential foundation of Arcturian techniques, reveals itself to be much more than a simple breathing exercise. It manifests as a refined practice of self-awareness and reconnection with the subtlest layers of existence. By intentionally directing attention to the act of inhaling and exhaling, the practitioner gradually silences the incessant flow of thoughts that cloud the mind, dissolving anxiety and patterns of restlessness that often keep the being trapped in fragmented realities. This act of observing, of feeling the air passing through the nostrils, expanding the lungs, and flowing back into the environment, serves as an anchor to the present, restoring the link between consciousness and the absolute now, where past and future lose their relevance and give way to full presence.

With the deepening of this practice, the body responds immediately. Each respiratory cycle, conducted with gentleness and full attention, triggers physiological and energetic mechanisms simultaneously. Deep, slow, and paced breathing promotes greater cellular oxygenation, revitalizing tissues and nourishing organs with pure energy, while the nervous system is enveloped by a subtle current of serenity. The heart rate slows down, adjusting harmoniously to the respiratory flow, and, in this rhythmic pace, muscle tensions dissolve almost as if by magic, allowing the very physical structure to reorganize itself in a state of deep relaxation and balance. This balance is not limited to the physical plane but reverberates through the emotional and mental layers, gradually dissolving the residues of stress accumulated in the fibers of body memory.

It is in this field of inner stillness that the true Arcturian alchemy begins to operate. The practice of cyclical breathing, one of the most precious transmissions of this cosmic wisdom, reveals itself as a key to accessing expanded states of consciousness and harmonizing the cerebral hemispheres. By inhaling deeply through the nose, the practitioner fills their internal space with a flow of light and air that, together, act as purifying and activating agents of the energy system. The conscious retention of breath, for a few seconds, allows this energy to spread through the inner layers, reaching points of stagnation and dissolving crystallized memories. The slow and prolonged exhalation through the mouth releases not only the physical air but also trapped emotional fragments, mental residues of repetitive patterns, and misaligned vibrational fragments.

The beauty of this technique lies in its flexibility and depth. With each cycle, it is possible to adjust the time of inspiration, retention, and expiration, according to the need of the moment and the area of the body or energy field that one wishes to work on. When there is a mental overload, for example, the retention time can be slightly extended, allowing the energy to concentrate on the skull and pineal gland, dissolving energetic congestion associated with excess thoughts. If the emphasis is on emotional release, the prolonged exhalation, accompanied by the conscious intention to release, leads to the gentle liberation of pain and anguish stored in the subtle layers of the being. This dialogue between breathing rhythm and conscious intention creates an internal field of self-transformation, where each breath is a sacred act of dissolving, reprogramming, and realigning.

Within this practice, the conscious visualization of the energy that accompanies each respiratory cycle acts as a catalyst for deep therapeutic processes. When inhaling, the practitioner is guided to visualize a white and golden light entering their body along with the physical air. This light is not an abstraction, but a living vibrational current, carrying Arcturian codes of harmonization and healing. It permeates every cell, every tissue fiber, every subtle circuit of the energy system, dissolving blockages and reactivating flows of vitality. When holding the breath, this light expands from the cell nucleus to the outermost layers of the energy body, as if each cell were a small sun radiating its own healing vibration.

At the moment of exhalation, the light that circulated internally expands beyond the physical limit, forming a sphere of vibrant energy around the practitioner. This sphere not only protects but also filters and refines the energy of the environment, allowing only frequencies compatible with internal harmony to be absorbed. It is in this continuous flow of inhalation, retention, and exhalation, permeated with light and conscious intention, that Arcturian breathing reveals its true potential: to be a bridge between the physical, emotional, and spiritual bodies, dissolving the boundaries between them until they recognize themselves as a single matrix of light in constant movement.

At certain moments of the practice, this visualization of light can be expanded to include the universal flow. The inhaled air is not just air – it is the cosmic breath that connects the individual to the living matrix of the universe. Each particle of cosmic prana carries not only vital energy but also encoded vibrational information, coming from the higher Arcturian spheres. This awareness transforms each inspiration into an act of communion with universal intelligence, where the individual receives guidance and vibrational alignment directly from the sources of cosmic light.

Among the most advanced practices, the tube of light breathing stands out, an energetic protocol for strengthening and protecting the auric field. When starting this practice, the practitioner visualizes a tube of white and golden light descending from the highest point of their consciousness – the crown – and passing through their entire central axis, until it anchors in the root chakra. This tube of light is, at the same time, a channel of reception and a protective shield. With each inspiration, the light descends from the cosmos, bringing codes of harmony and purification. With each exhalation, the light ascends from the earth, bringing vital force and stability. This ascending and descending flow, synchronized with the breath, establishes a continuous circuit of energization and protection, where the auric field is strengthened against external influences and harmonized internally.

The conscious practice of this tube of light creates an active vibrational shield, which not only blocks external interferences but also dissolves thought-forms and energetic fragments that may be attached to the auric field. It is as if the practitioner's own central axis were transformed into a column of living light, a pillar of connection between heaven and earth, where the personality and the soul meet in a single continuous flow of consciousness. This state of vertical alignment, sustained by conscious breathing and the visualization of the tube of light, generates a sense of security and cosmic belonging, where the being recognizes, in each breath, their place in the universal web.

Thus, each Arcturian breathing technique, from the simplest to the most advanced, forms part of a great map of return to the original state of fullness. Breathing then becomes an act of remembering – remembering who you are, remembering where you came from, and, above all, remembering that each breath, each pulse, is a unique note in the infinite symphony of creation. Conscious Arcturian breathing is not just a therapeutic or meditative practice; it is an invitation to become a co-author of your own vibrational reality, restoring, with each respiratory cycle, the sacred link between the individual essence and the living intelligence of the cosmos.

In the silence between each inspiration and expiration, the being finds their own primordial song – that unique frequency that pulses from before time and echoes far beyond form. Arcturian breathing techniques are not just paths to relaxation or to healing accumulated tensions, but living portals, where each conscious breath reveals the invisible bridge between matter and light, between mind and spirit. With each intentional respiratory cycle, the practitioner dissolves layers of forgetfulness, reinstalls the memory of their own original brilliance, and rediscovers, in the simplest and most vital act, that to breathe is to allow oneself to exist in full harmony with the cosmic pulsation, where the whole universe breathes together and returns, in the following breath, the soft echo of one's own eternity.

Chapter 11
Arcturian Hands-On Healing

Arcturian hands-on healing reveals itself as an energy healing practice deeply connected to the subtle realms of existence, transcending the mere technique of energy transmission. This approach, shaped and refined over millennia by the advanced wisdom of the Arcturians, is based on the understanding that the universe is woven by a vibrational matrix of living and intelligent energy, capable of responding to directed intention and awakened consciousness. Unlike traditional methods of energy healing, where the practitioner's personal energy may be used, Arcturian hands-on healing is anchored in the ability to serve as a pure and conscious channel for higher frequencies originating from the Arcturian collective consciousness, a consciousness that vibrates in tune with principles of universal harmony, unconditional love, and spiritual evolution. This connection between therapist, patient, and the Arcturian healing matrix forms a field of energetic coherence where the restoration of physical, emotional, mental, and spiritual health occurs in an integrated and dynamic way, respecting the unique rhythm of each being and promoting not only the relief of symptoms, but the real reorganization of the energy field in its entirety.

When applied, Arcturian hands-on healing is not limited to the simple action of placing hands on the physical body. It begins even before contact, through the internal preparation of the therapist, who aligns their vibrational frequency through meditation and specific invocations, adjusting their energy field to act as a bridge between the higher dimensions and material reality. This fine-tuning is essential to ensure that the channeled energy is pure, without personal interference or emotional distortions, allowing the Arcturian energy flow to freely travel through the therapist's subtle channels until it reaches the patient's auric field and energy centers. This energetic interaction creates a kind of "vibrational dialogue," where energy blockages, whether they originate from emotional traumas, limiting beliefs, or physical imbalances, are gently brought to the surface and realigned to the original matrix of balance. Thus, Arcturian hands-on healing acts not only as a tool for restoration, but as a catalyst for a broader process of self-recognition and reconnection with the primordial essence of each being.

The effectiveness of this practice lies in the fusion of three fundamental elements: clarity of intention, precision of visualization, and the solidity of the connection with the Arcturian consciousness. The conscious intention to heal functions as the vector that directs the Arcturian energy to the specific points that need attention, guiding the energy flow based on the real needs of the patient, which may transcend conscious perception. The clear and detailed visualization of energy, whether as light, crystalline flow, or vibrational waves, strengthens the field of action and creates a safe space for healing to occur, allowing the therapist to intuitively perceive where there is resistance or fluidity in the energy field. The connection with the Arcturian consciousness ensures that the process remains aligned with the highest frequencies available, providing not only healing, but also expansion of consciousness, spiritual insights, and the activation of latent potentials in the patient. This integration between intention, visualization, and connection makes Arcturian hands-on healing a multidimensional transformation tool, capable of promoting integral health and spiritual awakening in harmony with the cosmic principles of evolution and love.

  The application of energy through the hands, in Arcturian hands-on healing, manifests as a fluid and highly refined process of channeling cosmic life energy. The therapist, even before placing their hands on the patient's physical body, enters a state of deep attunement, where clarity of intention aligns with the opening of the energy channel. This inner preparation is fundamental, as it is through it that the therapist adjusts their vibrational frequency and consciously connects to the Arcturian healing matrix, becoming a pure conduit for the higher energy that flows directly from the Arcturian collective consciousness. It is not, therefore, a donation of the therapist's personal energy, but the conduction of a universal, immaculate flow that transcends individual limitations and carries with it the millenary wisdom of a civilization dedicated to harmony and spiritual evolution. During the process, the therapist visualizes, with crystalline precision, the Arcturian energy emerging from their hands in the form of pulsating light, translucent flows, or subtle vibrational waves, adjusting their perception according to the needs that the patient's energy field reveals.

This flow of energy is then directed to specific points on the body, guided by the therapist's intuitive perception and the energetic demands that present themselves subtly, but clearly, in the recipient's auric field. Each area of the body, each organ, each cell has a unique vibration, a particular energy signature, and the Arcturian energy, in its living intelligence, recognizes these signatures and adjusts itself in frequency and intensity, respecting the patient's integration limits. Arcturian hands-on healing, therefore, adapts organically to the vibrational reality of the one who receives it, permeating not only the physical level, but reaching the emotional, mental, and spiritual layers. Thus, localized pain can be relieved, inflammatory processes can be calmed, and organs or tissues in disharmony can be revitalized, not only by the energy influx, but by the reestablishment of the original matrix of balance that exists in the vibrational core of each being.

The technique, in its practical execution, consists of placing the hands gently on the affected area or at a small distance from the body, depending on the intuitive guidance received during the process. The hands become portals through which energy flows continuously, while the therapist maintains focus of consciousness and clarity of intention in restoring balance and internal harmony. The constant visualization of energy flowing like a luminous river or a vibrational breeze that penetrates the subtle layers, dissolves blockages, and revitalizes weakened structures, enhances the effectiveness of the technique. There is no rigidity in the positioning of the hands; they follow the natural contours of the patient's energy field, respecting their subtle anatomy and the vibrational information that is revealed as the energy travels through the internal pathways. This process not only restores health on physical and energetic levels, but also promotes the unblocking and purification of the chakras, restoring the natural flow of energy in the meridians and subtle networks that make up the human energy system.

Pure intention, sustained in thoughts and feelings harmonized with the greater purpose of healing, is one of the pillars that amplify the effectiveness of this technique. It is not just about desiring healing, but about anchoring the vibrational conviction that it is already underway, as an energetic reality that only awaits permission to manifest. This clear intention, when combined with a visualization rich in details – dancing lights, spirals of energy, or luminous mists permeating the patient's field – creates a safe and conducive vibrational environment for the integration of Arcturian energy. With each conscious breath, the therapist reinforces this field, allowing the energy to adjust precisely to the layers of cellular memory, crystallized emotional structures, and mental patterns that sustain imbalances. This loving and non-judgmental awareness, which perceives the being in its vibrational whole and not just in its diseased parts, allows the Arcturian energy to act not only as a remedy, but as a loving mirror, reflecting to the patient their own capacity for healing and self-recognition.

The connection with the Arcturian consciousness, in turn, is sustained by regular practices of meditation, visualization exercises, and specific invocations that tune the therapist to the higher frequencies of this collective consciousness. This connection is not an isolated event, but a bond cultivated over time, where the therapist becomes increasingly adept at recognizing and interpreting the flows of information and energy that are transmitted to them during the practice. In moments of greater sensitivity, it is possible for the therapist to directly perceive the presence of Arcturian beings or receive intuitive insights about the spiritual root of the symptoms presented by the patient. This interaction between dimensions, where the physical touch of the hands is united with the subtle guidance of the Arcturian consciousness, transforms each session into an act of energetic co-creation, where healing, learning, and spiritual expansion occur simultaneously.

In addition to physical and energetic restoration, Arcturian hands-on healing proves to be especially effective in unblocking and releasing repressed emotional content. The channeled energy acts as a vibrational key capable of accessing deep layers of the unconscious, where traumatic memories, denied emotions, and limiting beliefs are stored. By penetrating these fields, the Arcturian light gently dissolves the layers of resistance and pain, allowing the patient to access, understand, and integrate their emotions in a conscious and loving way. During the application, it is common for tears to arise, physical sensations to manifest, or old memories to surface spontaneously, signaling that the release process is underway. Hands-on healing on the head or heart region especially facilitates this work of emotional and mental healing, acting directly on the energy centers responsible for processing emotions and structuring thought patterns.

In this context, Arcturian hands-on healing becomes a powerful ally in the treatment of anxiety, depression, insomnia, and other mental disorders, offering not only symptomatic relief, but the possibility of reorganizing the vibrational field underlying these conditions. By placing the hands on the head, the therapist directs the energy to the subtle layers of the mind, dissolving dysfunctional thought fields, releasing accumulated tensions, and promoting a renewed mental clarity. This clarity does not arise merely as an absence of conflict, but as an expansion of perception, where the patient begins to see their experiences from new perspectives, freeing themselves from internal narratives that sustained patterns of suffering.

Arcturian hands-on healing also reveals itself as a path to strengthening spiritual connection and activating dormant potentials. By acting on the crown chakra, at the top of the head, the Arcturian energy resonates directly with the higher centers of consciousness, stimulating the opening of spiritual perception and the recognition of one's own divine essence. This process of spiritual reconnection is not forced, but facilitated by the loving presence of the Arcturian energy, which invites the patient to remember their cosmic origin and their active participation in the evolutionary flow of the universe. Spiritual traumas, ancestral vows, and karmic blockages can be dissolved in this process, making room for the being to express their light and inner wisdom in a freer and more authentic way. This spiritual activation, combined with physical, emotional, and mental healing, transforms each session into a portal of inner transformation, where the patient finds the golden thread that connects them to their greater soul purpose.

Thus, Arcturian hands-on healing transcends technique and reveals itself as a vibrational journey, where each touch, each flow of light, and each conscious breath are steps towards the reunion with the totality of the being.

Thus, each application of Arcturian hands-on healing unfolds as a silent dance between planes, where therapist and patient become co-authors of a healing process that is not limited to the relief of symptoms, but invites the re-signification of one's own existence. More than an energetic intervention, it is an invitation for the being, gently guided by the loving Arcturian intelligence, to return to its primordial center, where its luminous essence resides intact. In this space of deep recognition, the body aligns, the mind silences, the heart opens, and the soul remembers its wholeness, allowing healing to happen not as something imposed from the outside, but as a natural blossoming of what has always been present — the living memory of one's own balance, just waiting for the right light to awaken.

Chapter 12
Arcturian Psychic Surgery

Arcturian psychic surgery represents a highly refined spiritual technology, developed by an advanced civilization that deeply understood the interrelationship between consciousness, energy, and matter. Based on the premise that every physical imbalance is preceded by a disharmony in the subtle energy field, this technique acts directly on the vibrational layers that make up the energetic body, using highly precise frequencies to restore the harmonious flow of vital energy. Unlike conventional healing practices, which often focus on isolated physical symptoms, the Arcturian approach recognizes the human being as a multidimensional matrix, where emotions, thoughts, and spiritual experiences interact and shape overall health. The Arcturians, with their ancestral wisdom and their ability to operate in higher planes of consciousness, have developed methods that not only detect these subtle interferences before they solidify in the physical body, but are also capable of dissolving them with millimeter interventions, based on directed intention and cooperation with superior intelligences of the cosmic healing network.

The execution of this form of energetic surgery requires careful preparation of the therapist, who needs to elevate their own vibrational field to serve as a bridge between the Arcturian frequencies and the physical reality of the patient. This alignment is achieved through deep meditations, energetic purification processes, and a clear intention to serve the purpose of healing, free from judgments or personal desires. By establishing this state of attunement, the Arcturian therapist connects to a network of consciousnesses and spiritual technologies that operate outside the space-time limitations of the third dimension, allowing access to Akashic records, individual energy maps, and hidden layers of the patient's auric field. The intervention is then performed surgically, using light instruments shaped by the mind, such as vibrational blades capable of removing dense energetic adhesions, etheric plasma forceps to restructure broken energy filaments, and holographic reorganization fields that realign the original matrix of health and balance, as it exists in the higher planes of the being's consciousness.

Throughout the practice of Arcturian psychic surgery, communication between therapist, patient, and Arcturian consciousnesses is sustained by a constant telepathic flow, even if at unconscious levels. This communication field ensures that the intervention respects the patient's free will and the higher guidelines of their own evolutionary journey. The precision of the technique allows access to very specific layers of the energy system, from the removal of miasms and astral implants to the reintegration of soul fragments lost in deep traumas. Furthermore, the Arcturian action goes beyond mere symptom elimination, focusing on the global harmonization of the being, promoting reconnection with higher aspects of the patient's own consciousness. With this reintegration, the healing process is not limited to an isolated energetic repair, but activates a progressive realignment, leading the individual to a greater vibrational coherence and an expanded state of self-awareness and self-mastery.

The essence of Arcturian psychic surgery rests on a refined and deeply spiritual understanding of the origin of the diseases and imbalances that affect human beings. For the Arcturians, no physical manifestation arises in isolation or abruptly; any and every symptom or illness is only the final stage of a series of disharmonies that are rooted first in the most subtle levels of the energy field. These invisible layers, composed of vibrational flows that connect body, mind, and spirit, function as matrices that give shape and support to the integral health of the being. When this energetic web is compromised—whether by accumulated dense emotions, recurring low-vibration thoughts, or even external interferences such as miasms and astral implants—the integrity of this matrix weakens and the first signs begin to project onto the physical plane, gradually evolving into concrete symptoms and, eventually, into chronic or acute conditions.

The purpose of Arcturian psychic surgery is precisely to intervene in this process at the point where it originates, that is, in the energy field, before the dysfunctions crystallize as physical diseases. More than treating the visible effect, this technique is dedicated to identifying and correcting dissonant vibrational patterns, dissolving interferences, and restoring the original coherence of the vital flow. The precision and delicacy of these interventions allow not only the elimination of intrusive and harmful energies, but also the meticulous repair of damaged subtle tissues and the reconstitution of the energy structure in its integral and harmonious state. It is a spiritual technology of surgical refinement, capable of accessing deep layers of the being's vibrational anatomy and operating with millimeter accuracy, realigning the energy network that sustains physical, emotional, and spiritual health.

The beginning of this healing process requires careful preparation, both of the therapist and of the space in which the surgery will take place. The environment must be transformed into a true sacred space, a vibrational capsule that functions as a safe portal between dimensions. The creation of this environment begins with the energetic purification of the place, using techniques such as smudging with sacred herbs, high-frequency sounds, programmed crystals, and strategically placed protection geometries to seal the space against external interference. Each element is chosen and activated with the purpose of raising the vibration of the environment, making it a physical reflection of the harmony and serenity necessary for contact with the Arcturian consciousnesses.

Within this sacred space, the therapist begins their own internal preparation, which is just as essential as the preparation of the environment. Connection with the Arcturian consciousnesses is the foundation of the practice, and for it to occur in a pure and unobstructed way, the therapist must align their personal vibration with this elevated field of consciousness. This alignment is achieved through guided meditations that expand perception beyond the limits of the physical body, anchoring the mind in the timeless present where Arcturian frequencies can be accessed. In parallel, specific invocations are uttered, both mentally and aloud, not as pleas, but as sound keys that attune the therapist's vibration to the Arcturian light pattern. This tuning process is sustained by a clear and unwavering intention of healing, which must be expressed in a transparent way and free from any egoic expectation, functioning as a vibrational compass that guides the entire process.

With the environment sealed and the attunement established, the therapist turns their full attention to the patient. Before any intervention, it is essential to visualize the patient in their state of perfect health—a vibrational image where they are already free from any imbalance or interference. This visualization is not a mere fantasy or projection of desire; it is a vibrational coding that anchors the reality of healing in the quantum field, serving as an energetic matrix that will guide the reconstruction of the patient's field. Every detail of this image of wholeness is held in the therapist's mind as a possible reality and, above all, as an innate right of the being in the process of healing.

The execution of the surgery itself takes place through the direct manipulation of energy and light, using the mind as a surgical instrument and the hands as physical extensions of this intention. With a focused mind, the therapist sweeps the patient's energy field, scanning layer by layer until they locate blockages, densities, or subtle fragmentations. These zones of imbalance can manifest as dark spots, energetic knots, broken filaments, or even external structures, such as implanted energetic devices or parasitic accumulations. Each of these anomalies is carefully identified and recorded in the therapist's consciousness, who then begins the removal and repair.

The removal of blockages and implants is carried out by means of energetic telekinesis, where the therapist, in tune with the Arcturian frequencies, uses their own consciousness to move and dissolve the intrusive energies. Subtle light tools are visualized and used as needed—vibrational scalpels for precise cuts of harmful energetic connections, etheric forceps for extraction of implants, and flows of regenerative light to fill gaps left by the removals. With each movement, telepathic communication with the patient is maintained, even at an unconscious level, allowing the intensity and depth of the intervention to be adjusted according to the receptivity and individual needs of the being being treated.

This technique has a scope that goes far beyond the treatment of physical symptoms. Chronic pain, degenerative diseases, emotional traumas, spiritual blockages, and negative thought patterns can be accessed and treated through this methodology. Energetic tumors, crystallized emotional adhesions, and records of ancestral traumas are gently dissolved and released, while the essential vitality of the being is restored. Subtle organs and tissues receive direct vibrational repair, and the patient's original holographic matrix—the one that contains the record of their full health—is reactivated and reintegrated, allowing healing to flow from the energy field to the physical, from the inside out.

After the intervention, the recovery process is not limited to the energetic plane, but requires the patient's active participation in the integration of the new healing frequencies. Daily meditation, focused on visualizing the restored and vibrant field, allows the mind and body to gradually adjust to the new energetic configuration. Conscious breathing exercises help to anchor the frequencies and release emotional residues. Diet becomes an essential part of this process, with a focus on living, natural foods rich in vital energy. Physical movement, through practices such as yoga, walks in natural environments, and spontaneous dances, promotes circulation and adaptation of the new energy flow in the physical body.

In addition, creative and reflective habits, such as intuitive writing, artistic expression, and connection with activities that bring purpose and joy, become allies in maintaining the restored balance. Regular connection with nature and contemplative silence nourish the soul and reinforce the integration of the new vibrational matrix, while deep and restorative sleep ensures that the energetic updates are absorbed and stabilized at all levels of the being.

In this way, Arcturian psychic surgery expands far beyond a healing technique, becoming a conscious journey of vibrational realignment and rediscovery of the divine essence, where each adjustment and each release resonate as a silent invitation to the remembrance that true healing is, above all, the return to one's own cosmic nature.

In this flow of re-encounter, each session becomes a unique revelation, where the subtle layers of existence intertwine in a loving dialogue between personal consciousness and cosmic wisdom. It is in this territory without words, where the Arcturian light travels the hidden paths of the soul, that old wounds fade and new internal spaces open, preparing the being to inhabit their own light with more truth and wholeness. And so, under the invisible touch of this loving presence, healing ceases to be a destination and becomes a path, where each step reveals not only relief, but also the reminder that to be whole is, above all, to remember oneself as part of the Whole.

Chapter 13
Astral Travel and Distance Healing

Within the Arcturian perspective, astral travel and distance healing are configured as interdimensional practices deeply aligned with the expanded understanding of consciousness as the creative and expansive essence of being. By projecting consciousness beyond physical limitations, it becomes possible to access not only other planes of existence but also to act directly on the energy structures of people, environments, and situations, regardless of physical or temporal location. This ability to transcend three-dimensional space is not merely a mystical skill, but rather a refined spiritual technology, developed from the understanding that consciousness is the central axis that connects all realities, being the bridge between what is perceived as matter, emotion, thought, and spirit. The Arcturians, beings whose spiritual evolution has enabled them to operate fully in these expanded fields of existence, do not use astral travel only as a tool for exploration, but as a conscious mechanism of healing and realignment, capable of positively influencing the energetic weavings that sustain health, evolution, and existential harmony of the beings with whom they come into contact.

In this context, the conscious projection of the astral body is understood as a natural act of unfolding consciousness, which temporarily frees itself from the physical anchor to access higher vibrational layers. This separation is not an escape or a disconnection from the material plane, but rather an expansion of the field of perception, allowing the practitioner to act as an agent of healing and harmonization on multiple layers simultaneously. Preparation for Arcturian astral projection involves not only relaxation and visualization techniques, but a consistent vibrational elevation, achieved through ethical alignment, clarity of purpose, and attunement to the higher spheres of Arcturian consciousness. This expanded state of consciousness allows the traveler to perceive their own energy in a more refined way, recognize disharmonious vibrational patterns in themselves and others, and directly access sources of wisdom and healing that transcend the linear limits of time and space. In this way, astral travel becomes an act of conscious service, where the loving intention of healing is conducted by Arcturian vibrational currents, configuring a continuous flow of restorative energy that acts directly on the subtle fields of the recipient of healing.

The practice of distance healing within this perspective, therefore, is not limited to a simple energetic emission or sending of good intentions. It occurs as a surgical and highly targeted process, where the astrally projected therapist connects directly to the vibrational matrix of the patient, whether incarnate or discarnate, and clearly identifies the blockages, fragments, and energetic distortions that require realignment. This connection occurs in a telepathic and vibrational field that dispenses with physical presence, as Arcturian consciousness recognizes that distance is only an illusion created by the linear perception of the human mind. Arcturian distance healing, by acting directly on the energy matrix, is able to catalyze processes of physical, emotional, and spiritual regeneration simultaneously, always respecting the free will and evolutionary moment of each being. The combination of conscious astral projection with the transmission of healing frequencies creates a field of resonance that not only treats isolated symptoms, but harmonizes the overall energy field of the being, promoting reconnection with their higher essence and opening paths for their evolution and self-realization.

The projection of consciousness, considered the first and fundamental step for the full realization of Arcturian astral travel, begins with a process of gradual decoupling between the astral body and the physical body. This separation does not occur abruptly or forced, but as a subtle and progressive unfolding, where consciousness learns to float between the two states of presence — sometimes immersed in physicality, sometimes expanded in the etheric layers that transcend material density. This detachment, although natural to the soul, requires from the practitioner a refinement of internal perception, a sensory recognition of their own energy, and the ability to identify the exact moment when the physical anchor is released, allowing the astral body to rise.

To achieve this state of conscious detachment, the practitioner is invited to immerse themselves in deep relaxation techniques, where each muscle and each thought are gently dissolved, like mist dissipating at dawn. The comfortable posture, either lying down or in a semi-reclined position, favors complete relaxation. Breathing becomes a guiding thread, a measured rhythm that subtly refines mental waves and opens space for immersion in deeper layers of one's own interiority. Each inhalation brings awareness of presence, and each exhalation releases the tensions of the day, opening the internal field for the out-of-body experience.

In this expanded state of relaxation, the practice of visualization becomes an essential key. The practitioner begins to visualize their astral body, initially as a silhouette of translucent light, which rests perfectly on the physical body, like a second skin of pulsating energy. Gradually, this luminous silhouette begins to detach from the dense form, as if levitating gently, separating by centimeters, then by meters, until it is perceived floating above the physical body, but still connected by a thin silver cord — the energetic link that preserves the safety of the soul in transit.

This practice of visualizing astral separation is not just an induction tool, but a training that strengthens the clarity of perception. The more the practitioner exercises this visual and energetic displacement, the greater their ability to recognize the real moment of separation becomes. Regularity, patience, and persistence are fundamental components of this process, as each attempt consolidates the subtle pathways that connect waking consciousness to astral consciousness, making the transition increasingly fluid and natural.

Once detached, the Arcturian astral body is conducted beyond the three-dimensional sphere, entering vibrational planes where the density of matter gives way to the plasticity of light. Arcturian astral travel, far from being a simple excursion between dimensions, is a journey guided by a clear intention and a precise attunement to the vibrational coordinates of the planes one wishes to access. Among these planes, the astral plane itself stands out, where emotional energy and the Akashic records intertwine in mutable landscapes, mirroring both collective projections and individual memories.

Further up, there is the mental plane, a sphere of existence where thoughts take shape and ideas condense into geometric structures that reveal the underlying architecture of reality. On this plane, the Arcturian traveler can clearly access the web of beliefs that sustain their perception of existence, as well as identify and dissolve limiting patterns that operate as barriers to the expansion of consciousness. Beyond it, the causal plane is revealed, where the primordial causes, the vibrational seeds that originate events and experiences, can be recognized and reprogrammed. This plane is like the cosmic womb where intention and vibration create the matrices that will later unfold in the denser planes of manifestation.

The richness of these dimensions is not limited to passive contemplation. Arcturian astral travel is, above all, an opportunity for encounter and interaction with spiritual guides — Arcturian consciousnesses, ancestral mentors, and beings of light who act as facilitators of the evolutionary journey. These encounters not only offer teachings and revelations, but serve as vibrational mirrors, reflecting to the traveler their own essential light and their shadow areas still not integrated.

Another essential aspect of this practice is the possibility of directly accessing information about past lives. By entering the Akashic records, the traveler can revisit crucial moments of their multidimensional trajectory, understanding the origins of certain emotional patterns, karmas, or latent gifts. This access, conducted with responsibility and guided by Arcturian consciousness, reveals itself as a powerful tool for self-knowledge and healing.

But it is at the intersection between astral travel and distance healing that the Arcturian practice reveals its deepest therapeutic potential. During conscious projection, the traveler can direct their attention to beings, environments, or situations that need energetic realignment. Arcturian consciousness understands that the energy of healing is not restricted to physical proximity, as the vibrational matrix that sustains each being is accessible from any point in the universe.

The process of Arcturian distance healing begins with the creation of a sacred space, a protected vibrational field where the connection with Arcturian consciousness is established in a clear and safe way. This space, supported by geometries of light and Arcturian frequencies, functions as an interdimensional bridge between therapist and patient. The clear definition of intention is the foundation of this bridge: the therapist expresses their purpose verbally and mentally, visualizing the patient enveloped in a field of golden or blue light, representing their state of perfect health.

The practice continues with the direct telepathic connection to the patient's vibrational matrix. This connection is not an invasion or manipulation, but a loving and respectful attunement, where the therapist, acting as a channel, captures information about blockages, fragments, or distortions in the patient's energy field. This vibrational reading is accompanied by a continuous flow of healing energy, which is transmitted directly from Arcturian consciousness to the patient's field, dissolving obstructions and reactivating natural flows of vitality.

This distance healing can be applied to a wide range of conditions: from chronic pain and degenerative diseases to emotional traumas and spiritual blockages. Each condition is perceived not only as an isolated symptom, but as a reflection of disharmonies in multiple layers of the being. The goal of Arcturian healing is not to suppress symptoms, but to restore the overall harmony of the energy field, allowing the organism itself, in its physical, emotional, mental, and spiritual dimensions, to rediscover its natural state of balance and fulfillment.

Ethics is a non-negotiable guideline in this process. Before any intervention, the patient's informed consent is obtained, ensuring that they understand the process, its benefits, and its possible limitations.

Confidentiality is preserved at all stages and the therapist's responsibility includes the constant search for improvement and the recognition of the importance of collaboration with other health professionals, especially in cases where multidisciplinary intervention is necessary.

Thus, Arcturian astral travel and distance healing become not only practices of energetic intervention, but expressions of a loving and conscious service, where the expansion of perception and the activation of inner light go hand in hand. By integrating technique, ethics, and elevated purpose, the Arcturian therapist not only facilitates healing processes, but acts as a guardian and catalyst for the essential remembrance that each being is, in its origin, light, harmony, and love in full expression.

In this interweaving of dimensions, Arcturian astral travel and distance healing reveal themselves as subtle and profound expressions of the principle of unity, where no pain, imbalance, or fragment of consciousness exists isolated from the greater whole. Each incursion into the subtle planes is not only an act of assistance to the other, but a luminous mirror that returns to the therapist the perception of their own vastness and cosmic belonging. By serving as a bridge between worlds and consciousness, they understand that to heal is to remember — to remind the assisted being of their integral and luminous essence, and to remind themselves of the greater purpose of their presence here and now: to be a channel for the light that never extinguishes and the compassion that permeates all planes of existence.

Chapter 14
Energy Cleansing and Protection

Energy cleansing and protection are fundamental pillars for preserving a being's vibrational integrity, functioning as continuous practices of sanitization and strengthening of the subtle bodies amidst the constant energy exchanges that occur in daily life. Every human being, in their multidimensional nature, is not just a physical organism, but a complex structure of energetic layers that interact directly with the environment, with other beings, and with invisible planes of existence. This energy field, or aura, acts as a sensitive membrane that captures, processes, and emits frequencies, reflecting internal and external states. However, this vibrational porosity also makes the field susceptible to impregnations, fragmentations, and imbalances originating from dense emotions, dissonant thoughts, and external influences. Understanding this vulnerability, the Arcturian civilization developed an extensive and refined knowledge focused on maintaining energy purity and resilience, recognizing that vibrational clarity is indispensable not only for health but also for fluid connection with higher planes of consciousness.

The practice of Arcturian energy cleansing transcends simplified approaches and is based on principles that align conscious intention, connection with universal currents of light, and the application of specific vibrational technologies, all calibrated to act directly on the most vulnerable points of the auric field. In its purest form, energy cleansing consists of dissolving emotional residues, crystallized thought-forms, and energetic fragments incompatible with the soul's original vibration, returning the field to its natural malleability and luminosity. Arcturian techniques involve the creation of polarized light flows, which traverse each layer of the energy field with surgical precision, identifying and neutralizing any dissonant vibrational records. This process can be enhanced through the activation of internal portals, located in the main energy centers, allowing the elimination of miasms directly to multidimensional transmutation fields, where these energies are recycled into their primordial form. In addition to removing impurities, Arcturian cleansing activates the soul's original vibrational memory, restoring alignment with the essential codes of health, balance, and innate protection.

Energy protection, in turn, does not consist merely of erecting defensive barriers, but of developing a vibrational structure so coherent and luminous that it acts as a self-regulating field, naturally repellent to incompatible frequencies. Instead of creating rigid walls, the Arcturians teach that true protection arises from the full integration of the being with their own essence and with the higher currents of light. This constant connection activates a dynamic vibrational shield, adaptable to circumstances and sensitive to the subtleties of the environment. This shield is not a layer isolated from the being, but a conscious extension of their own energetic presence, accurately reflecting the level of internal coherence and active spirituality. Arcturian techniques include encoding the energy field with high-frequency geometric patterns, such as golden light tetrahedrons, blue plasma spheres, and multifaceted crystalline meshes, which not only filter external influences but also continuously reprogram the field, adjusting its frequencies to resonate exclusively with forces compatible with the individual's evolutionary journey. By uniting cleansing and protection as complementary and continuous practices, the being not only preserves their energetic integrity but also expands their capacity for conscious interaction with subtle realities and their connection with guides, mentors, and higher spheres of cosmic intelligence, sustaining their evolution in a safe, harmonious, and fluid manner.

The first step to establishing efficient energy protection lies in the deep cleansing of the subtle field, a process that begins with the systematic removal of negative, intrusive, or dissonant energies accumulated both by internal factors and external influences. These impregnations can arise from recurring thoughts of a pessimistic nature, repressed emotions that crystallize in the energy body, dense environments where disharmonious vibrations overlap in invisible layers, or even through draining interactions with people whose energy load tends to be absorbed, often unconsciously, by those who have more sensitive and permeable fields.

In this context, the creative and conscious visualization of white and golden light reveals itself as a fundamental technique, acting as a conducting thread of the cleansing by projecting, with clarity and intention, a luminous current that traverses all layers of the aura. This light, endowed with vibrational intelligence, acts as a subtle solvent, penetrating the points where the energy appears dense or opaque, dissolving accumulations and dismantling hardened thought-forms. White light carries primordial purity, while golden light adds the frequency of spiritual wisdom and solar protection, uniting cleansing and safeguarding in a single continuous flow.

To enhance this process, one can resort to smudging with consecrated herbs, an ancestral technique that combines the power of intention with the accumulated plant wisdom in the subtle realms of nature. White sage, rosemary, rue, or palo santo, when burned slowly, release not only their characteristic aroma but also a specific vibration that spreads through the environment and penetrates the aura, loosening and eliminating low-frequency impregnations. The smoke acts as a bridge between the planes, guiding the misaligned energies out of the personal field and returning them to the earth for transmutation.

In addition to light and herbs, purifying crystals are invaluable allies in this process. Stones such as black tourmaline, capable of absorbing and neutralizing intrusive energies, or smoky quartz, known for its power to transmute negative charges into neutral frequencies, can be strategically positioned around the body or held in the hands during the cleansing practice. At the end of the process, these crystals must be properly discharged and purified, either in running water, sunlight, or earth, so that they are ready for further action.

Complementing the arsenal of techniques, the application of purifying essential oils adds an extra layer of care, combining the aromatic power with the healing frequency of plants. Rosemary oil, known for its protective and energizing action, or lavender, whose gentleness is capable of enveloping the aura in a film of serenity, can be applied to strategic points on the body, such as wrists, neck, and chest, or diluted in water for spraying in the environment. This practice, in addition to strengthening the natural energy barrier, creates a field of well-being that makes it difficult for new forms of dense energy to adhere.

The effectiveness of this entire cleansing sequence lies not only in the mechanical execution of the techniques but above all in the regularity with which they are practiced and the quality of mindfulness and directed intention that permeate each gesture. When the being becomes aware of their own energy field and takes active responsibility for its preservation, cleansing transcends the punctual character and transforms into a continuous state of self-observation and vibrational refinement.

From the purification of the field, it becomes natural to establish a second level of energy security: the conscious creation of a protective shield. This shield is not a rigid or impermeable barrier, but an intelligent vibrational membrane, capable of selecting and filtering which energies can approach and which are automatically repelled. The first technique for building this shield involves the clear and detailed visualization of a luminous layer enveloping the entire body and expanding beyond the aura, like a second skin of light.

This protective layer can take different forms according to personal affinity or the specific need of the moment. It can be visualized as an egg of golden light, which reflects and repels dense energies, or as a translucent sphere that pulsates in harmony with the breath and adjusts its density according to the quality of the environment. Some practitioners, especially those with developed visual sensitivity, prefer to create a faceted shield, composed of small mirrors of light that reflect and fragment any dissonant frequency that tries to approach.

Again, crystals play an important reinforcing role in sustaining this shield. Protective stones, such as black obsidian, tiger's eye, or blue kyanite, can be carried as amulets or placed in the four corners of a space, forming a vibrational network that stabilizes and strengthens the existing protection. These crystals, by acting in resonance with the conscious intention of the practitioner, become physical anchors of an essentially energetic process.

Similarly, essential oils with protective properties can be incorporated into the practice, not only for their aroma but also for the subtle frequency they emit. Cedarwood oil, with its root and stability energy, is especially useful for protecting the energy field from external intrusions, while frankincense, traditionally associated with spiritual practices, creates an atmosphere of sacredness that naturally repels interference. These oils can be used in diffuser necklaces, added to room sprays, or applied directly to the skin, always with proper dilution.

The sustenance of this energy shield depends not only on the techniques applied but also on the clarity with which the intention is declared. Verbally expressing, aloud or mentally, the intention to protect one's own field and define the desired energy boundaries imprints a personalized vibrational programming on the shield. This declaration of energy sovereignty acts as a direct command to the field, informing it about which frequencies are welcome and which will be immediately dissolved or reflected.

The continuous practice of these protection techniques, combined with sensitive perception and self-observation, forms a dynamic layer of security, which not only repels dense energies but also adjusts its density and permeability according to the need of each situation. In safe and elevated environments, the shield can become more subtle, allowing for greater energy exchange; in challenging situations, it automatically densifies, reinforcing the protective barriers.

However, even before the application of any technique, there is an indispensable preliminary step: the conscious identification of negative and intrusive energies. This recognition occurs not only through diffuse sensations but through the development of intuitive perception, cultivated through meditation and the practice of mindfulness. By silencing the mind and expanding inner listening, the being learns to subtly perceive variations in their own field, identifying regions of anomalous density or vibrational oscillations that indicate the presence of external influences.

At the same time, careful observation of one's own physical body and emotional and mental states serves as an alert panel, directly reflecting the quality of energy interaction. Symptoms such as persistent fatigue without apparent cause, sudden emotional swings, or recurring intrusive thoughts may indicate the presence of dissonant energies or energetic fragments that have attached to the field. This early identification allows cleansing and protection techniques to be applied before these energies take root and create deeper blockages.

Thus, cleansing and protection are not isolated or sporadic practices, but continuous expressions of a state of conscious presence, where each technique naturally integrates into the being's spiritual and energetic routine, ensuring not only the maintenance of vibrational integrity but also the full blossoming of the luminous essence that inhabits each subtle field.

In this way, energy cleansing and protection, from the Arcturian perspective, cease to be understood as reactive responses to external interference and become sacred practices of self-care and vibrational sovereignty. Each gesture of purification and safeguarding becomes an act of recognition of one's own value and the sacredness of existence, reaffirming the awareness that each being is the legitimate guardian of their energetic temple. By cultivating this vigilant and loving posture, where the zeal for one's own field reflects respect for one's own evolutionary journey, the human being strengthens as a luminous and conscious presence, capable of transiting through subtle and dense worlds without losing their essential spark, sustaining themselves as a point of integral light amidst the vastness of existence.

Chapter 15
DNA Rebalancing

DNA rebalancing, as understood and applied by the Arcturians, is based on the expanded view that the human genetic code is much more than a biological sequence restricted to dense matter. DNA is, in the Arcturian perspective, a living spiral of light and information, acting as a vibrational bridge between the physical body and the subtle fields of higher consciousness. Each strand contains encoded records of past experiences, ancestral patterns, and unrealized potentialities, composing a dynamic matrix that responds directly to intention and energetic interaction. Through advanced spiritual technologies, the Arcturians have developed the ability to access these hidden layers of DNA, where information resides not only about physical health but also about the spiritual evolution of the soul in its multidimensional trajectory. This approach allows going beyond mere correction of genetic mutations or cell regeneration, paving the way for the activation of dormant sequences that contain the original codes of perfection and spiritual sovereignty of humanity.

The Arcturian approach to DNA rebalancing involves a precise combination of directed intention, holographic visualization, and manipulation of extremely high-frequency vibrational fields. The trained therapist, acting as a conscious channel of this technology, connects to the patient's original matrix of perfection, a kind of energetic blueprint that exists in the higher planes of consciousness, even before physical incarnation. This primordial template serves as a reference to identify deviations, fragmentations, or blockages inserted throughout the evolutionary journey, whether by emotional trauma, ancestral inheritances, environmental influences, or artificial energetic implants. Once the point of imbalance is identified, the Arcturian therapist directs flows of encoded light to the DNA, dissolving the distortions and rewriting the genetic information based on the original vibration of the soul. This process not only promotes the restoration of physical health but also releases crystallized emotional patterns, allowing the being to resume its natural flow of expression and manifestation.

In addition to repairing damage and removing inherited patterns, one of the main objectives of Arcturian DNA rebalancing is the activation of the so-called light codes. These codes are vibrational segments present in multidimensional DNA, responsible for storing the higher potentialities of the soul, including psychic abilities, creative talents, connection with higher spheres of consciousness, and the ancestral memory of stellar civilizations of which the being is a part. Many of these codes are inactive or partially blocked due to the vibrational density of the physical plane and the energetic interferences accumulated over successive incarnations. By activating them, the healing process expands beyond the physical body and the emotional field, promoting a true reintegration of fragmented consciousness, restoring the full flow between the Higher Self and the incarnated personality. This awakening of latent potential transforms the individual into a conscious channel of their own divinity, capable of co-creating their reality in a more harmonious way and aligned with the purpose of their soul.

The understanding of the influence of Arcturian energy on the structure of human DNA starts from the expanded conception that this subtle helix of life and memory does not end in its chemical and molecular sequences visible to the eyes of conventional science. For the Arcturians, DNA is a vibrational field in constant dialogue with higher dimensions of consciousness and the cosmic spheres from which the soul originates. Its physical structure, composed of nucleotides and chemical bonds, is only the densest face of an infinitely more complex energetic web. This multidimensional mesh encompasses filaments of encoded light that extend beyond the physical body, connecting directly to the subtle bodies, planetary grids, and stellar memory libraries. In this context, DNA is much more than a mere inherited biological program: it is a living receptacle of information, a transmitter of spiritual potentialities, and a vibrational mirror where the state of the soul is reflected and manifested.

Among the most precious elements of this vibrational structure are the so-called light codes, energetic segments that remain, for the most part, latent or partially dormant. These codes are vibrational records inserted in the core of the genetic spiral, containing information about gifts, innate abilities, stellar memories, and spiritual potentialities specific to each being. However, due to the vibrational density of the Earth and the successive layers of conditioning, trauma, and energetic manipulations accumulated over countless incarnations, most of these codes remain inaccessible to ordinary consciousness. The activation of these luminous records is, therefore, an essential step not only for the restoration of integral health but also for the reconnection of the soul with its original wisdom and its full capacity for conscious manifestation in the physical plane.

The process of DNA reprogramming, as applied by the Arcturians, constitutes an advanced spiritual technology that operates precisely on this subtle interface between biology and higher consciousness. Unlike traditional interventions that are limited to correcting genetic mutations or cell regeneration at purely physical levels, this technique works directly on the vibrational layers of DNA, restoring its original flow and reintegrating information and potentialities that have been fragmented or blocked. Reprogramming begins with the conscious connection between the therapist and the patient's vibrational field, establishing an energetic bridge between the soul's original matrix of perfection and the current genetic expression of the incarnated being. This original matrix, preserved in the Akashic records and in the higher layers of the spiritual field, contains the divine plan of the being, free from distortions and interferences.

With the clear intention of restoring this alignment, the Arcturian therapist initiates a process of holographic visualization, where the patient's DNA is projected in its luminous form, a pulsating spiral of light permeated by strands of colored energy and geometric codes. This visualization is not merely symbolic but a true access to the living records contained in the quantum field of the being. From this projection, the therapist, acting as a conscious channel of Arcturian technology, uses their own mind and energy field to manipulate and reorganize the flows of light and information that make up the subtle DNA. Each distortion, each fragment crystallized by ancestral traumas or by external influences, is identified and gently dissolved through the emanation of specific frequencies of encoded light.

This energetic manipulation, often described as a form of vibrational telekinesis, does not involve any physical contact, as it happens in the subtle levels of the vibrational matrix. Guided by higher consciousness and the direct assistance of the Arcturians, the therapist adjusts the frequencies of the DNA until its resonance harmonizes with the original plan of the soul. This adjustment allows not only the repair of structural damage and the removal of limiting genetic patterns but also the progressive activation of dormant light codes. Each activated code is like a key that unlocks internal portals, releasing flows of information and potentialities that were sealed, awaiting the moment of their conscious reactivation.

The effectiveness of this technique rests fundamentally on two pillars: pure intention and clarity of visualization. Consciousness, understood as a creative force, is the primordial element that shapes the vibrational reality of the being. Therefore, the therapist's intention is not just a mental statement, but a vibrational emanation that aligns their own energy matrix with the patient's original matrix of perfection. Likewise, the holographic visualization of DNA in its whole and luminous state serves as an energetic model, a kind of vibrational map that guides and anchors the reprogramming process. When the conscious mind, loving intention, and Arcturian light converge in a single flow, the DNA responds, reorganizing itself according to the matrix of perfection and reactivating the segments that had been disconnected or obscured.

The regular practice of meditation and conscious visualization is encouraged not only as a complement but as an integral part of this process of rebalancing and reprogramming. Through constant practice, the patient learns to access and interact with their vibrational field, becoming an active agent of their healing and evolution. With each visualization, the bond with the original matrix strengthens, and the conscious perception of their own luminous nature expands, facilitating the dissolution of limiting beliefs and inherited conditioning.

The benefits of Arcturian DNA rebalancing extend far beyond physical healing. This technique has proven effective in the treatment of genetic and degenerative diseases, deep emotional traumas, limiting ancestral patterns, and energy blockages of various natures. By repairing damage to the subtle structure of DNA and releasing crystallized records, the process strengthens the immune system, rejuvenates cells, and restores harmony between body, mind, and spirit. At the same time, the activation of light codes promotes the expansion of consciousness and reconnection with inner wisdom, allowing the incarnated being to reclaim forgotten talents, latent psychic abilities, and a clearer understanding of their life purpose.

With each activated code, a new layer of perception unfolds, revealing ancestral information about the being's stellar lineage and its role within the vast cosmic web. The activation of these records is not merely informative but transformative, as each fragment rescued from stellar memory expands individual consciousness and strengthens the direct connection with the higher spheres of guidance and protection. The progressive awakening of these potentialities becomes, therefore, a process of reintegration of the soul with itself, dissolving the veil of forgetfulness that separated it from its true origin and its essential mission.

In this context, the practice of Arcturian DNA rebalancing transcends personal healing, becoming a true journey of cosmic reconnection. Each being who reclaims their light keys and reintegrates their original matrix of perfection contributes to the vibrational upliftment of the collective, radiating their restored light to the planetary field and assisting, directly and lovingly, in the global awakening of humanity. Thus, human DNA ceases to be a simple biological inheritance and reveals itself, at last, as what it really is: a living library of light and memory, a bridge between worlds, and a master key to the full manifestation of the divine in the physical plane.

In this continuous process of rescue and reintegration, Arcturian DNA rebalancing reveals itself as a profound invitation to rediscover the true spiritual identity, dissolving layers of forgetfulness that have accumulated over eras and recalibrating the being so that it can express, without distortions, the original melody of its soul. Each vibrational adjustment, each activated light code, not only unlocks latent potentialities but also returns to the individual the remembrance of their direct connection with the stellar webs and the divine intelligence that pulses in each cell. Thus, DNA ceases to be just a hidden record and begins to vibrate consciously as a song of cosmic belonging, where each reconnected strand of light remakes the links between the human, the divine, and the expanding universe.

Chapter 16
Treatment of Chronic Diseases

The Arcturian approach to treating chronic diseases establishes a broad and integrative paradigm that considers the human being as a complex unit of physical body, conscious and unconscious mind, emotions, and soul in constant interaction with the energetic universe around them. This holistic view is based on the principle that no chronic disease arises in isolation or randomly, but rather as a result of an accumulation of energetic imbalances, unresolved emotional traumas, crystallized mental patterns, and disconnection from one's own spiritual essence. Each physical manifestation, whether it be persistent pain, organic dysfunction, or cellular deterioration, is understood as a direct reflection of more subtle layers of disharmony that settle throughout the individual's life trajectory, often rooted in ancestral experiences or even in records of past lives. For the Arcturians, curing a chronic disease requires much more than combating its visible symptoms—it requires the willingness to dive deep into the patient's inner universe, unveiling the hidden messages that the physical body expresses through pain and limitation.

This healing process begins with a careful investigation of the individual's vibrational history, analyzing the significant events of their biography, their recurring beliefs and behaviors, their unprocessed emotional memories, and the energetic patterns inherited from their family lineage. Chronic disease, from the Arcturian perspective, is seen as the culmination of a cumulative process, where the natural flow of vital energy is gradually interrupted by layers of fear, guilt, resentment, and spiritual disconnection. This energetic blockage manifests first in the subtle bodies—the emotional body, the mental body, and the etheric body—and, over time, densifies until it reaches the physical body, generating chronic inflammation, tissue degeneration, metabolic disorders, and immune weakening. Therefore, restoring full health means, first and foremost, removing these layers of disharmony and restoring the free and harmonious flow of vital energy, so that each cell of the body can vibrate in resonance with the greater purpose of the incarnated soul.

The Arcturian approach therefore understands that every chronic disease is also an opportunity for awakening and spiritual evolution. Far from being just a condition to be eliminated, chronic illness is interpreted as a call from the soul for the individual to review their life choices, reframe their emotional pain, reorient their thoughts, and reclaim their sacred connection with their own essence. This spiritual healing process does not exclude conventional medical care, but transcends it by integrating it with vibrational therapies, belief reprogramming, release of traumatic memories, and reconnection with the primordial source of love and wisdom that inhabits each being. True healing, in this expanded view, is not just the remission of physical symptoms, but the reintegration of the individual to their multidimensional totality, where body, mind, and spirit dance in harmony, allowing life to flow with ease, health, and purpose.

The Arcturian approach to the treatment of diseases such as cancer, diabetes, and arthritis integrates harmoniously with conventional medicine, understanding that both approaches, when combined with intelligence and sensitivity, offer the patient a much broader and more effective field of possibilities for the restoration of health. Conventional medicine, with its vast range of diagnostic tools and pharmacological treatments, is recognized for its ability to identify biological changes with precision and act directly on inflammatory, infectious, and degenerative processes. Through laboratory tests, high-resolution images, and biochemical markers, it is possible to monitor the evolution of the disease in real time and adjust interventions according to the response of each organism. Antibiotics, anti-inflammatories, immunomodulators, and hormone replacement therapies make up only a fraction of the therapeutic arsenal that modern science makes available, often bringing immediate relief and preventing the aggravation of structural and functional lesions.

However, the Arcturians teach that this direct care of the physical body, although valuable and necessary in many cases, needs to be complemented by a broader vision, capable of encompassing the energetic and emotional layers that, ultimately, sustain and influence pathological processes. Therefore, complementary therapies play a central role in the Arcturian integrative proposal, offering ways to restore energy flow, dissolve vibrational blockages, and awaken the cellular memory of balance and self-regulation. Acupuncture, by stimulating specific points in the meridians, reestablishes the circulation of vital energy and harmonizes the organic systems globally. Homeopathy, in turn, acts on the vibrational level of matter, sending subtle stimuli that invite the organism to rediscover its original point of balance, respecting its individuality and its healing rhythm. Phytotherapy, through the judicious use of medicinal plants, harnesses the biochemical intelligence of nature to nourish, purify, and regenerate tissues, while nutritional therapy adjusts the diet to provide the essential nutrients that support cellular health and rebalance the biological terrain where the disease has settled.

The integration between these approaches, which might seem complex or conflicting in a fragmented view, becomes fluid and synergistic when guided by the Arcturian principle that each being is unique and their healing process must be equally unique. The development of an individualized therapeutic plan is the result of an active collaboration between doctors, therapists, and, above all, the patient themselves. Open communication between the professionals involved ensures that every aspect of the being is taken into consideration: physical symptoms, mental patterns, crystallized emotions, inherited traumas, and karmic cycles that reverberate in the current experience. This continuous dialogue allows interventions to be adjusted according to the body's response and the evolution of consciousness, transforming the treatment into a journey of self-discovery and empowerment.

Arcturian medicine contributes uniquely to this integration by decoding the energetic blockages and limiting beliefs that, often in a hidden way, feed the manifestation of the disease. Through vibrational readings and subtle mappings, it is possible to identify in which areas of the patient's energetic field the vital energy has been interrupted, which traumatic memories are stored in the cellular layers, and which unconscious patterns sabotage the body's spontaneous regeneration. Chronic disease, from this expanded perspective, is no longer seen as an isolated event and is understood as the final expression of a long trajectory of disconnection and suffering, calling not only for medicines and technical procedures, but for acceptance, listening, and reframing.

In this context, diet and lifestyle emerge as fundamental pillars of healing. The physical body, being the final receptacle of all energetic, mental, and emotional influences, needs to be properly nourished to support the processes of cleansing and regeneration. A diet based on whole, minimally processed, fresh, and vital energy-rich foods offers the body not only nutrients but vibrational information that reverberates in the cellular field. Colorful fruits, organic vegetables, whole grains, seeds, and nuts form the basis of a living nutrition, which not only feeds the body but communicates messages of harmony and vitality to each cell.

For patients undergoing healing processes for chronic diseases, a specific dietary protocol is recommended, adjusted to individual needs. Each morning, one can start the day with a green juice.

Throughout the day, light and balanced meals are prioritized, avoiding ultra-processed foods, refined sugars, and hydrogenated fats. Vegetable soups with turmeric and garlic, colorful salads with extra virgin olive oil and sunflower seeds, and dishes with quinoa, chickpeas, and medicinal mushrooms are examples of preparations that deeply nourish without overloading the digestive system.

Parallel to diet, lifestyle needs to be adjusted to create an internal and external environment conducive to healing. Regular physical exercises, adapted to the patient's physical condition, help to mobilize toxins, strengthen muscles, and stimulate energy circulation. Walks in contact with nature, yoga or tai chi practices, and conscious stretching promote the balance between movement and relaxation, while daily meditation offers a safe space for encountering oneself and the more subtle aspects of one's own essence.

The quality of sleep is equally crucial. Deep rest is the moment when the physical body performs cellular repairs, processes vibrational information received during the day, and reconnects with the cosmic flow of regeneration. Creating a peaceful nighttime routine, with reduced artificial stimuli, use of aromatherapy with lavender or chamomile essential oils, and conscious breathing practices before bed, facilitates entry into deep states of rest and healing.

In addition to physical and energetic care, emotional and spiritual well-being is supported by activities that nourish the soul. Creative expressions such as painting, writing, or dancing offer channels for the release of repressed content and the rediscovery of innate talents. Connection with nature, whether through forest bathing, contemplation of the sea, or cultivating a garden, reconnects the human being with their primordial essence. Seeking meaning and purpose in each stage of the journey, even in moments of pain and uncertainty, transforms the disease into a teacher and the cure into a reconciliation with one's own history.

This deep dive into the hidden layers of the disease is supported by the identification of the root causes, an essential step in the Arcturian approach. By investigating not only symptoms and laboratory tests, but also thought patterns, repressed emotions, and transgenerational traumas, the energetic and emotional matrix that sustains the pathology is revealed. Understanding these roots allows for the development of a truly curative treatment plan that not only silences symptoms, but removes their original sources.

Finally, the restoration of energetic balance is consolidated through specific vibrational techniques: the laying on of hands to realign chakras, acupuncture sessions to unblock meridians, personalized homeopathic formulas, and aromatic baths for auric cleansing. Each technique, applied with intention and sensitivity, strengthens the integrity of the energy field and allows the light of the soul to flow freely again, dissolving the accumulated shadows and restoring health as a reflection of inner harmony.

Healing, in this context, ceases to be a final goal and transforms into a dynamic state of continuous reconnection, where each step taken towards self-knowledge reverberates directly in the health of the body and the clarity of the soul. The patient's journey, conducted with love and respect for their singularities, reveals itself as a process of rescuing not only physical vitality, but the very spiritual memory of integrity and belonging to the universal flow of life. Thus, chronic disease, once seen as a relentless adversary, takes on the role of a silent teacher, leading the human being to the encounter of what is most true in itself: its innate capacity to create, regenerate, and dance in harmony with the cosmos and with its own divine essence.

Chapter 17
Mental and Emotional Health

Arcturians understand mental and emotional health as a direct reflection of the internal harmony between mind, emotions, and energy field, where every thought and feeling reverberates not only in the physical body but in all the subtle layers of being. Mental and emotional disorders, such as anxiety, depression, and persistent traumas, do not arise in isolation nor can they be reduced to simple chemical imbalances. They represent external manifestations of profound misalignments that originate in the disconnection between the individual and their spiritual essence, in the accumulation of poorly processed emotional experiences, and in the perpetuation of limiting mental patterns. This vision expands the concept of mental health, understanding that true emotional and psychic stability is only achieved when the consciousness of the human being aligns with their inner truth and with the natural flow of cosmic energy that permeates all existence. In this context, the Arcturians develop therapeutic approaches that access deep layers of the psyche, release blockages rooted in past lives, correct energy distortions, and reprogram the vibrational patterns that sustain dysfunctional mental and emotional states.

The treatment process involves an expanded listening of the individual's vibrational field, where each recurring thought, each repressed emotion, and each limiting belief is identified as a specific frequency that can be harmonized or transmuted. This energetic listening allows us to understand that mental and emotional disorders are not mere responses to external events, but rather results of a long history of internal conditioning, reinforced by traumatic memories, frustrated expectations, and disconnection from one's own divine essence. Chronic fear, for example, is perceived as a vibration of contraction that, if maintained, interferes with the free circulation of vital energy, weakens the nervous system, and compromises mental clarity. Likewise, depression reflects an energy depletion that results from disconnection with the soul's purpose, with creativity, and with the natural flow of consciousness expansion. Understanding the energetic pattern underlying each disorder is the first step to dissolving the vibrational matrix that sustains it, allowing new, higher, and more harmonious frequencies to reorganize the energy field and promote emotional and mental balance.

Arcturian healing, therefore, is not limited to isolated techniques, but is a continuous process of reconnection with the divine essence that inhabits each being. Meditation is used as a tool for daily vibrational adjustment, helping the mind to slow down and tune in to the frequency of peace and harmony that permeates the higher planes. Creative visualization allows direct access to the subconscious, reframing painful memories and replacing dense mental images with internal scenarios of healing, lightness, and reconnection with one's own inner light. DNA reprogramming techniques go beyond biology, acting on the energy field to deactivate ancestral records of suffering and activate the light codes that restore psychospiritual harmony. By integrating these practices with the conscious recognition of emotions and with the gradual release of emotional and mental conditioning, the individual not only heals their disorders but is reborn in a new consciousness, where mental and emotional health ceases to be a distant goal and becomes a natural expression of their connection with the whole.

The Arcturian techniques aimed at treating anxiety, depression, and other mental and emotional disorders constitute a sophisticated set of practices that, in essence, seek to restore the vibrational alignment of the individual, promoting integration between mind, emotions, and energy field. Among these techniques, meditation occupies a central role. More than a simple relaxation exercise, it is understood as a bridge that connects the ordinary consciousness of the mind to the subtle space of peace, where the divine essence of the being can be heard. By dedicating themselves to meditative practice, the individual gradually silences the incessant noise of compulsive thoughts and worries fueled by the conditioned mind, allowing deeper layers of silence and lucidity to settle in. In this space of inner stillness, the nervous system slows down, cortisol levels balance, and a deep sense of inner security emerges. This security is the basis for repressed emotions to come to the surface without causing collapse or retraction, being welcomed as part of the natural flow of existence. The regular practice of meditation thus becomes a vibrational anchor, helping the mind to tune in more and more to the frequencies of harmony, peace, and confidence that emanate from the higher planes of consciousness, gradually dissolving the vibrational fields associated with anxiety and chronic fear.

Complementing meditation, creative visualization is used as a tool for deep reprogramming of the subconscious mind. Unlike a simple fantasy or daydream, visualization is conducted with precision, guiding the individual to construct highly symbolic mental images charged with therapeutic intention. Through it, the mind is led to abandon internal landscapes marked by fear, scarcity, or pain, replacing them with luminous, expansive, and harmonious scenarios, where the being itself is seen and felt in its fullest and healthiest state. This conscious replacement of internal images creates new neural pathways and, above all, restructures the vibrational matrix of the mental field. By visualizing themselves as healthy, serene, and connected to their inner light, the individual emits vibrational signals consistent with this desired reality, attracting it to their physical and emotional experience in an increasingly consistent way.

A technique especially valued by the Arcturians is DNA reprogramming. This practice is based on the understanding that human DNA is not only a biochemical structure that encodes proteins but also a receiver and transmitter of vibrational frequencies linked to ancestral memory and the spiritual lineage of each being. Traumatic experiences lived by past generations, fears and beliefs inherited from ancestors, and vibrational records of pain accumulated over successive lives form layers of distortions in the field of energetic DNA. Arcturian reprogramming acts directly on these subtle layers, deactivating the vibrational records of suffering and activating the light codes that correspond to the full potential of the being. This process occurs in an expanded state of consciousness, where the individual's own higher presence, in communion with the Arcturian guides, identifies the records to be transmuted and reframed. As these pain codes are dissolved, the neural synapses related to patterns of fear, self-sabotage, and disconnection are weakened, opening space for the creation of new neural connections aligned with joy, confidence, and clarity of purpose. Thus, DNA reprogramming not only acts on the energetic sphere but also has a direct impact on the functioning of the brain and nervous system, restoring harmonious communication between body, mind, and spirit.

Within this approach, past life therapy represents an even deeper dive into the vibrational roots of mental and emotional disorders. The Arcturians understand that many of the phobias, anxieties, depressions, and patterns of self-sabotage experienced in the present are echoes of unresolved experiences in other incarnations. Fragments of pain, fear, or guilt frozen in vibrational records of the past remain active in the energy field of the being, influencing their choices, emotions, and automatic reactions in current life. By accessing these records under the safe guidance of trained therapists or directly with Arcturian assistance, the individual has the opportunity to revisit these memories, understand them in light of their evolutionary journey, and, above all, release the imprisoned emotional charge. This release not only dissolves the current symptom but also deeply reorganizes the individual's energy grid, allowing flows of vital energy previously blocked to circulate freely again.

This integrative approach, which combines meditation, visualization, DNA reprogramming, and past life therapy, reflects the Arcturian understanding that each mental or emotional symptom is just the tip of a much deeper vibrational iceberg. Therefore, true healing can only occur when the individual is led to explore and harmonize their most subtle layers, recognizing themselves as a multidimensional being whose emotions, thoughts, and experiences transcend linear time and the simple current biography.

Within this context, the importance of emotional balance is continuously emphasized as a fundamental pillar for integral health. Emotions, far from being just automatic responses to external stimuli, are understood as direct vibrational messages from the soul, signaling where there is flow and where there is blockage in the energy field. Emotions such as anger, fear, and sadness, when repressed or crystallized, create true energetic knots, which limit the free circulation of vital energy and manifest in the physical body in the form of chronic muscle tension, hormonal changes, and organic imbalances. On the other hand, emotions such as joy, love, and gratitude promote vibrational expansion, strengthen the immune system, and create an energy field of positive attraction, where experiences aligned with well-being flow naturally.

On this path of healing and expansion, the practice of self-observation becomes an indispensable tool. Observing oneself without judgment, welcoming each emotion that emerges without rejection or repression, recognizing one's own automatic mental patterns and understanding their origins allows the individual to stop being hostage to their unconscious emotional reactions. This lucid self-observation, combined with the constant practice of acceptance and healthy expression of emotions, creates an internal environment where transformation becomes possible.

For this transformation to consolidate, the Arcturians emphasize the need to deeply investigate the emotional history of each individual. This investigative dive, conducted in therapeutic sessions, ranges from the analysis of current symptoms to the mapping of repetitive behavior patterns, limiting beliefs, childhood traumas, and dysfunctional family dynamics. This investigation is not merely analytical, but energetic and vibrational, allowing the true root of the disorders to be identified and understood within an expanded perspective of the being's evolutionary journey.

The restoration of emotional balance, in turn, is supported by a vast range of energy healing techniques.

Laying on of hands, acupuncture, aromatherapy, and crystal therapy are just some of the tools used to dissolve blockages, harmonize flows, and strengthen the energy structure as a whole. When vital energy returns to flowing without obstacles, cellular health is restored, the nervous system is strengthened, and chronic inflammatory processes are softened or even eliminated.

Finally, this entire journey culminates in the promotion of inner transformation. More than stopping symptoms, this transformation is understood as the realignment of the being with their soul purpose, where each challenge, each crisis, and each repressed emotion become steps towards the rediscovery of one's own divine potential. When this reconnection is consolidated, mental and emotional health ceases to be a distant goal and becomes the natural expression of a being who lives in peace with themselves and in harmony with the cosmic flow of existence.

In this process of rescuing mental and emotional health, the individual not only frees themselves from the invisible chains that imprisoned them to old pains but also rebuilds their own perception of who they are, recognizing themselves as a vast consciousness in constant evolution. Each layer dissolved, each memory reframed, and each emotion welcomed expands the internal space for the light of the true essence to radiate with more strength and clarity. Thus, the mind ceases to be a battlefield and emotion, a territory of fear or lack of control; both become allies in the creation of a reality more coherent with the truth of the soul, where inner balance is reflected in healthier relationships, more conscious choices, and a deep trust in the loving intelligence that sustains existence.

Chapter 18
Pain Treatment

Pain, in the Arcturian perspective, is understood as a sophisticated communication mechanism between the different bodies of the human being—physical, emotional, mental, and spiritual—signaling the existence of blockages, disconnections, or deep imbalances that need to be recognized and integrated. More than an isolated symptom or a localized biological response, pain is seen as a tangible manifestation of the interruption in the free flow of vital energy, reflecting accumulated tensions, crystallized traumas, and repressed emotions that lodge in specific regions of the body. Each painful point carries encoded information about the individual's experiences, their unprocessed memories, and the degree of misalignment between their higher consciousness and their daily choices. When treating pain, Arcturians do not limit themselves to immediate relief, but investigate its hidden meaning, transforming it into a key to access deeper layers of the psyche and soul, where the true roots of suffering can be found and transmuted.

This integrative approach is based on the premise that pain is a multidimensional phenomenon, arising from the constant interaction between the physical, energetic, and emotional levels. Chronic pain in the lower back, for example, may reflect not only physical overload or postural misalignment but also an emotional overload related to feelings of helplessness, financial insecurity, or fear of losing control of one's life. Similarly, recurring migraines may point not only to dietary or hormonal factors but to an internal conflict between the rational mind and intuition, or to excessive self-demand and creative repression. By identifying these hidden layers of meaning, Arcturian therapists understand that pain is not an enemy to be fought, but rather an ally that reveals the internal paths that cry out for attention, care, and realignment. In this process, sensitive and compassionate listening to the body becomes an essential therapeutic practice, allowing pain to cease to be seen as a punishment or a failure and to be recognized as an opportunity for transformation and expansion of consciousness.

To promote this transformation, Arcturian techniques combine refined energetic approaches with practices of spiritual reconnection and vibrational reprogramming. The laying on of hands acts directly on the subtle fields, dissolving dense accumulations of stagnant energy and restoring the harmonious flow of vital force along the meridians and energy centers. The use of crystals is applied specifically, choosing stones whose frequencies resonate with the vibrational needs of each individual, amplifying energy cleansing and strengthening the points of greatest vulnerability. Essential oils, selected according to the predominant emotional vibration, are used to create aromatic healing fields that harmonize breathing, relax the nervous system, and induce deep states of well-being. Through guided meditation and creative visualization, the individual is invited to dialogue with their pain, understanding it as a portal to self-awareness and self-realization. This internal dialogue allows not only physical relief but the loving integration of fragmented aspects of the psyche, promoting a healing that is, at the same time, cellular and spiritual, punctual and expansive, freeing the being to experience their existence with more lightness, fluidity, and alignment with their soul purpose.

Arcturian techniques for relieving physical and emotional pain are not limited to punctual or superficial interventions but delve into a broad understanding of the being, addressing pain as an invitation to rebalance and reintegrate the disconnected parts of the human experience. Among the most used practices in this context, the laying on of hands occupies a central place, being considered a direct form of communication between the therapist and the individual's energy fields. With the palms facing the affected area, the hands become conscious channels for healing energy, directing specific vibrational flows that dissolve blockages, relieve tension, and activate cell regeneration. This subtle yet potent contact creates a high-frequency magnetic field where physical matter and subtle energy meet to restore lost harmony. The therapist, acting as a mediator between dimensional planes, tunes into the patient's unique vibrational signature and thus directs energy not only to the manifested pain but also to its underlying causes, promoting relief that is at the same time physical, emotional, and spiritual.

In addition to the laying on of hands, energetic acupuncture emerges as a refined technique, adapted from the traditional knowledge of oriental medicine, but elevated to a practice that acts directly on the vibrational flows and the energetic architecture of the being. In this approach, acupuncture points are stimulated without the need for physical needles. Instead, finger pressure or even crystalline instruments of high vibrational purity are used, which gently touch the skin or are held at a certain distance, while conducting subtle flows of energy to the corresponding meridians. The stimulation of these strategic points unblocks congested channels, allowing the vital energy to return to its natural flow, thus reducing pain and promoting an immediate sensation of relief and lightness. Each point touched or energized acts as a gateway to memories and emotions that, once recognized and welcomed, release naturally, dissolving tensions accumulated over years.

In parallel, energetic massage is applied as a way to reconnect the physical body with its original vibrational matrix. Unlike conventional massage, which acts directly on the muscles and tissues, energetic massage combines gentle touches with conscious directions of healing energy. The therapist's hands glide slowly over the skin or just hover a few centimeters from the body surface, while following the subtle maps of the auric field and meridians. This combination of physical touch and etheric touch releases muscle tension, but also loosens layers of emotional protection and dissolves crystallized traumas. The body, understood as a sacred receptacle of memories and experiences, responds to these touches with a progressive relaxation that is not only muscular, but profound, reaching the emotional and spiritual levels. Thus, the feeling of well-being that emerges is not only due to physical relief, but also to the recognition and release of repressed emotional content, which has long sought expression.

Crystals, in turn, are introduced as amplifiers of therapeutic intention and as powerful allies in restoring vibrational balance. Each crystal is chosen with precision, taking into account not only the physical pain presented but also the energetic and emotional nature associated with it. Persistent pain in the lower back, for example, can be treated with hematite or black tourmaline, crystals known for their ability to ground and dissolve dense accumulations of fear and insecurity. Pain in the solar plexus region, often associated with emotional tension and excessive self-criticism, can be worked with citrine or amber, stones that radiate warmth, confidence, and emotional fluidity. The crystals are placed directly on the skin, along the chakras, or in specific geometric patterns around the body, creating healing grids that modulate the vibrational frequency of the entire auric field. This subtle and profound interaction between body, emotion, and vibration allows the being itself to recognize and reorganize its internal energies, promoting healing that starts from the core of its consciousness and expands to the physical body.

Complementing this healing ecosystem, essential oils are used as carriers of ancestral plant frequencies, capable of directly accessing the emotional layers and cellular records of the body. Each oil is selected based on the nature of the pain and the emotions associated with it. For pain related to nervous tension and accumulated stress, lavender is often chosen for its ability to calm the nervous system and create an environment of internal security. For pain associated with repressed anger or blocked frustrations, peppermint essential oil can be used, offering freshness and immediate energy unblocking. The oil is diluted in gentle vegetable bases and applied directly to the skin, with circular and loving movements, or diffused in the environment, creating aromatic atmospheres that envelop the patient in layers of invisible healing. By inhaling the aromatic molecules, the limbic system is activated, facilitating emotional release and the reframing of painful memories.

The essence of this Arcturian approach lies in the understanding that each pain is a unique vibrational story, which must be heard and honored before being dissolved. Therefore, the treatment is never standardized or mechanical, but shaped from the sensitive listening of the body and soul of each being. Physical pain may have roots in evident physical traumas—falls, injuries, past surgeries—but also in subtle processes of disconnection from the soul's purpose or in tensions accumulated over years of emotional repression and self-abandonment. Similarly, emotional pain is understood as a vibrational response to unintegrated experiences: unprocessed losses, self-deprecating beliefs, disharmonious relationships that have left deep impressions on the energy field. Each of these pains, whether physical or emotional, is investigated at its origins, not to be fought or silenced, but to be recognized as a messenger that points to what needs love, care, and attention.

From this deep understanding, the treatment plan is elaborated in a completely individualized way, considering not only the symptoms presented, but the complete vibrational history of the being. The therapist, guided by their sensitivity and connection to the Arcturian frequencies, conducts each session as a compassionate dive into the patient's inner universe, where the techniques—laying on of hands, energetic acupuncture, subtle massage, crystals, and essential oils—are not ends in themselves, but instruments to restore the interrupted dialogue between body, mind, and soul. Each touch, each aroma, each energetic pulse rescues a forgotten part of one's own essence, gathering scattered fragments and reintegrating them into the original matrix of harmony and wholeness. In this space of loving listening and deep reconnection, pain ceases to be an enemy or an obstacle, and becomes recognized as a sacred bridge to one's own healing, inviting the being to return to its center and rediscover its own essential light.

Thus, the treatment of pain, from the Arcturian perspective, transcends the mere search for immediate relief and reveals itself as a portal of self-knowledge, where each physical or emotional discomfort is transformed into an invitation to reconciliation with oneself. Pain, when welcomed with respect and deep listening, loses its rigidity and opens the way for the vital flow to resume its natural course, allowing the body, mind, and soul to dance in harmony again. Each dissolved layer, each honored memory, and each released emotion reconstructs the inner map of the being, restoring not only the sought-after relief but the living memory of its own capacity for self-healing, reconnection, and rebirth in new levels of consciousness and wholeness.

Chapter 19
Women's Health

Women's health is understood by the Arcturians as a reflection of the dynamic harmony between the physical body, emotions, mind, and spiritual energy, where each biological cycle represents a sacred portal of transformation and self-knowledge. Hormonal, menstrual, gestational, and menopausal processes are seen not only as physiological functions but as living mirrors of a woman's deep connection with the rhythms of the Earth, the tides, and cosmic flows. Each phase of a woman's life is recognized as an opportunity to access subtler layers of inner wisdom, unveiling hidden aspects of the soul and strengthening the link between her earthly body and her divine essence. In this sense, women's health goes far beyond the absence of symptoms or the maintenance of reproductive functions, encompassing the ability to fully live one's cyclical nature, honoring hormonal fluctuations as messengers of one's emotional and spiritual needs, and recognizing one's womb as an energetic center of creation, healing, and transformation.

The Arcturians understand that every discomfort or imbalance that arises in the female body is a coded message, inviting the woman to turn inward and listen to the whispers of her ancestral soul. Persistent menstrual pain, for example, may carry memories of ancestral repression of femininity or repressed emotions related to self-expression and sexuality. Infertility may be linked to unconscious beliefs of inadequacy or deep-seated fears of welcoming the creative energy of life. The symptoms of menopause, in turn, reflect not only the biological transition but also the invitation to release patterns of self-judgment, deconstruct rigid identities, and embrace the wisdom of the elder, connecting with one's spiritual lineage and with planetary cycles. Instead of treating these symptoms as biological failures or isolated problems, the Arcturian approach integrates them into the larger process of awakening feminine consciousness, allowing each phase of a woman's life to be a portal of healing and expansion.

Arcturian therapeutic practices for women's health combine energy harmonization techniques with rituals of inner connection, always respecting the uniqueness of each woman and her evolutionary moment. The laying on of hands on the energy centers of the womb and heart dissolves vibrational blockages, restoring the flow of vital energy between the uterus and heart — an essential connection for a woman to manifest her creativity, fertility, and personal power. The use of specific crystals, such as moonstone for hormonal regulation or rose quartz for strengthening self-love, amplifies the healing capacity of one's own energy field. Essential oils, combined in vibrational synergies, act as sensory portals to release cellular memories and promote reconnection with the intuitive wisdom of the body. In addition, therapeutic writing, intuitive dance, and women's circles create sacred spaces of welcome, where experiences of pain, pleasure, fear, and empowerment can be shared and reframed. In this way, women's health becomes a sacred path of return to one's own center, where awareness of cyclical energy is transformed into an internal compass for deep healing, spiritual blossoming, and the manifestation of one's purpose on Earth.

The way the Arcturians understand and assist women's health in its different life phases is deeply connected to the cyclical view of existence, where each stage carries not only physiological challenges but also invitations to access specific layers of self-knowledge and spiritual awakening. In puberty, when a girl's body begins its dance with the lunar rhythms and opens itself to hormonal language, the Arcturians offer practices that help harmonize the intense chemical and emotional fluctuations that accompany this period. It is a phase of discovering one's own bodily identity and connection with feminine ancestry, and the Arcturians understand that the way this passage is experienced leaves deep energetic imprints that influence the woman's entire journey.

In this phase, energy harmonization is applied with extreme delicacy, always respecting the young woman's emotional vulnerability and sensory intensity. The laying on of hands is often performed on the heart center and the womb, uniting these two energetic poles and allowing the young woman to feel safe in her transforming body. This practice not only dissolves blockages formed by fears or insecurities but also invites the girl to listen to the intuitive voice that inhabits her womb, cultivating from an early age a relationship of respect and affection with her cycles. Alongside this, grounding practices are recommended, such as direct contact with nature, especially with natural waters — rivers, seas, or lakes — where she can symbolically surrender her doubts and fears, allowing the waters to flow and renew her energy.

In addition to energy harmonization, self-esteem is carefully nurtured through creative practices. The Arcturians value spontaneous writing, where the young woman is encouraged to record her perceptions and emotions, as if she were writing letters to her own body. This writing acts as a bridge between the conscious mind and the unconscious layers, helping her to name and welcome her new sensations. Free dances, without rigid choreography, are also encouraged. Moving intuitively, allowing the body itself to create gestures and rhythms, helps the young woman feel comfortable in her own skin, gradually dissolving the shame or strangeness that can emerge when faced with her new curves and flows.

As the young woman begins to live with her menstrual cycles, the Arcturians guide practices that help transform menstruation from a physiological event into a conscious rite of passage. Creating small rituals, such as lighting a candle and offering a prayer to her own womb or creating a lunar diary to record the cycle along with her emotions and dreams, helps establish an intimate connection with this sacred flow. This positive relationship with menstrual blood helps prevent, from an early age, distortions about her body and her femininity, promoting self-esteem rooted in acceptance and cyclical power.

When a woman enters adulthood, and her relationship with her body, fertility, and pleasure becomes even more complex, the Arcturian approach expands to address specific challenges of this phase. Issues such as menstrual irregularities, premenstrual tension (PMS), endometriosis, and infertility are treated not only as biological dysfunctions but as reflections of energetic and emotional blockages that emerge to be welcomed and reframed. The laying on of hands continues to be an essential practice, directed with greater emphasis to the ovaries and uterus, allowing cellular memories to be released and the flow of creative energy to be restored.

Arcturian acupuncture, adapted to the vibrational frequencies they recognize in the female meridians, is applied to unblock specific channels linked to reproductive energy and creative expression. In sessions where the woman is comfortably lying down, small crystals are positioned over the acupuncture points, functioning as energy amplifiers, while Arcturian therapists use soft mantras to harmonize the subtle flows of the body.

Aromatherapy assumes a crucial role in this cycle, with synergies carefully chosen for each need. To regulate the cycle and relieve PMS, for example, a mixture of geranium, clary sage, and lavender essential oils is recommended. The use is simple and should be integrated into the routine: in an amber glass bottle, mix 50 ml of grape seed vegetable oil with 5 drops of geranium, 4 drops of clary sage, and 3 drops of lavender. This mixture can be gently massaged into the lower abdomen daily, especially during the premenstrual days, or used as an oil for immersion baths, where warm water enhances absorption and emotional release.

In pregnancy, the Arcturian approach values the deep connection between mother and baby, understanding that this subtle telepathic communication begins from conception. Energy harmonization sessions are aimed at strengthening this bond, helping the mother to listen to the baby's needs and adjust her own energy to create a loving and safe uterine field. Crystals such as rhodochrosite, rose quartz, and carnelian are often used to create energy grids around the womb, while aromatic baths with sweet orange and chamomile oil help relieve tension and strengthen the intuitive bond with the baby.

Upon entering menopause, a woman crosses a threshold of profound transformation, where her physical and energetic body undergoes a recalibration to integrate the wisdom accumulated throughout life. The Arcturians see this phase as the crowning of the feminine journey, a moment where the woman, by releasing biological fertility, is invited to channel her creative energy into her spiritual and community expression. Hot flashes, insomnia, and mood swings are understood as signs that vital energy is being redirected to new centers and new forms of creation.

The recommended practices for this phase include the laying on of hands on the heart center and the pineal gland, helping the woman to integrate her new vibrational frequency and connect with her expanded spiritual vision. Aromatherapy for menopause includes synergies such as clary sage, fennel, and peppermint essential oils, which can be used in environmental diffusers to create a field of freshness and clarity. The basic recipe consists of 100 ml of distilled water in a spray bottle, with 8 drops of clary sage, 5 drops of fennel, and 5 drops of peppermint. This mist can be used throughout the day, especially when hot flashes occur.

Intuitive dance and women's circles become especially valuable at this time of life, as they offer a safe space for women to share their experiences and reframe their mature bodies as temples of wisdom. Rites of passage, where older women share their stories and symbolic offerings are made to the earth, help to anchor this new identity with reverence and joy.

Regardless of the phase of life, the Arcturians remind us that the key to women's health is loving listening to the body and conscious celebration of each cycle. When a woman understands that her womb is a living portal of wisdom and that each symptom is a message, she ceases to fear her transformations and learns to dance with them, integrating pain and pleasure as equally sacred parts of her spiritual and physical journey.

On this sacred path of reconnection with her cyclical essence, the woman rediscovers that her health is not a fixed state or a distant goal, but a living dance between her shadows and lights, between her vulnerabilities and powers. Each pain embraced, each emotion released, and each cycle honored weaves the invisible thread that connects her to all the women who came before her and those who are yet to come, forming a great web of ancestral and collective healing. By finding herself again as the guardian of her own creative energy and as the embodied expression of feminine wisdom, the woman recovers not only her physical and emotional balance but also deep confidence in her intuition, her voice, and her power to give birth not only to lives but to entire realities aligned with the truth of her soul.

Chapter 20
Child Health

Child health, from the Arcturian perspective, is understood as a dynamic process in which the child's body, mind, and spirit harmoniously adjust to their journey of incarnation and learning on Earth. From birth, each child carries a unique vibrational field, composed of ancestral records, past life memories, and the essential purity of their spiritual essence. This subtle field, extremely sensitive, interacts with the environment, absorbing energetic impressions, emotions, and external stimuli, which directly influences their physical, emotional, and spiritual development. For the Arcturians, child health is not just the absence of disease, but the preservation of the child's energetic integrity, allowing their inner light, natural curiosity, and creative potential to flourish freely, without the vibrational and emotional burdens that tend to accumulate during childhood when their subtle needs are not recognized.

Based on this expanded understanding, promoting child health involves creating high-frequency energy environments where the child feels safe, respected, and free to express their true essence. The emotional bond with parents and caregivers is seen as a fundamental vibrational bridge, as the child, especially in the early years, regulates their own energy field in tune with the field of those around them. Any tension, fear, or emotional imbalance in adults is perceived and assimilated by the child, influencing their energetic stability and, consequently, their health. Therefore, the Arcturian approach encourages the practice of loving and conscious presence by parents, cultivating moments of full connection, in which the child feels seen, heard, and welcomed in their authenticity. This energetic and emotional listening allows the child to trust their own intuitive flow, strengthening their self-esteem and their innate capacity for physical and emotional self-regulation.

In addition to the environment and family ties, the child's connection with nature is considered an essential pillar for their healthy development. Contact with natural elements—earth, water, air, fire, and the plant and animal kingdoms—directly nourishes their energy field, anchoring their soul in the physical plane in a light and harmonious way. Children, according to Arcturian wisdom, have a spontaneous connection with the energy flows of the Earth and the cosmos, and this connection is strengthened whenever they play outdoors, touch the earth, feel running water, or observe the cycles of the moon and the sun. This energetic exchange with nature not only strengthens their immune system and physical vitality but also nourishes their psychic and spiritual sensitivity, allowing them to naturally develop their subtle perceptions, creativity, and self-healing capacity. By integrating these cares with energy harmonization techniques, such as laying on of hands, harmonization with crystals, and the conscious use of therapeutic aromas, it is possible to support each child in their growth in an integral way, respecting their uniqueness and providing the necessary resources for their body, mind, and spirit to evolve in balance and fullness.

    The Arcturian approach to the health of babies and children recognizes that each phase of child development requires sensitive and attentive listening, capable of capturing not only physical needs but also the emotional, energetic, and spiritual vibrations that permeate the experience of growth. From the first days of life, babies are seen as souls newly anchored in the physical plane, whose bodies still vibrate in a subtle and ethereal frequency, close to their spiritual origin. In this context, the bond with the parents is understood as a kind of conducting wire, a vibrational bridge that helps the baby's soul to feel safe, welcomed, and anchored in its new bodily reality. This connection, more than just physical, is deeply energetic and emotional, and each touch, each loving look, and each whispered word carries the ability to harmonize the baby's subtle field, helping them to adjust more serenely to the density of matter and the rhythm of incarnation.

    To strengthen this primordial bond, the Arcturian approach suggests daily practices of conscious presence, where parents or caregivers offer the baby moments of skin-to-skin contact, silent affection, and intuitive communication. During breastfeeding or cuddling moments, parents are invited to breathe deeply, harmonize their own emotions, and, with a serene mind, intentionally send vibrations of love, security, and welcome. This simple, yet powerful practice has the effect of calming the baby's nervous system, promoting more restful sleep and an overall state of relaxation and confidence in the new environment around them.

In the first months of life, it is also recommended to create a vibrationally pure environment, where the presence of soft sounds, natural lights, and delicate aromas contributes to the baby's serenity. Crystals such as rose quartz, amethyst, and selenite can be discreetly positioned in the baby's room, preferably near the crib, forming a kind of protective and harmonizing field. A warm water immersion bath with a few drops of chamomile or lavender is indicated to relax the body and subtly align the energy flows, especially after days when the baby has received many visitors or experienced more intense stimuli.

As the child grows and enters the preschool phase, the Arcturian approach broadens its view, understanding that this is the stage in which the soul, already a little more rooted in the physical body, begins to explore its own expression in the world. Self-esteem, understood as the child's confidence in their own inner light, becomes a central axis of care. It is in this period that the first spontaneous creative expressions—such as free drawing, intuitive dance, and imaginative play—need to be encouraged and recognized as legitimate expressions of the child's essence. Every creative expression is, for the Arcturians, a direct extension of the soul's vibrational field, a kind of energetic language that needs to be respected and valued.

To foster this creative and emotional blossoming, it is recommended that caregivers set aside daily moments to play with the child without directing or correcting, just accompanying and celebrating their spontaneous creations. It is important to create spaces in the routine where the child can freely paint, model clay, invent stories, and interact with their toys or natural elements, such as leaves and pebbles collected on walks. This space of creative freedom helps the child develop self-confidence, recognize their intrinsic value, and learn, from an early age, to trust their intuitive perceptions, which are fundamental for their emotional self-regulation.

In this same phase, the child's emotional body begins to interact more directly with the social and family environment, which can generate moments of frustration, fear, or insecurity. To support the child's emotional balance, the Arcturian approach recommends the practice of small sessions of laying on of hands, done by the parents or caregivers themselves, with the following guidance:

Invite the child to lie down comfortably.

Play soft and serene music, preferably nature sounds or high-frequency instrumental melodies.

Breathe deeply and intend love and calm.

Place your hands, one on the center of the child's chest (heart chakra) and the other on the forehead (frontal chakra).

Remain like this for a few minutes, just emanating love and security, without words or corrections.

End the moment with a hug and words of encouragement.

This simple harmonization technique helps to dissolve accumulated emotional tensions, promoting a sense of deep acceptance and vibrational security.

When the child reaches school age, the Arcturian approach also focuses on supporting the balance between mind, body, and vibrational field in the face of new learning and socialization demands. The school environment, with its rules, stimuli, and interactions, represents a new and challenging energy field, which can, in some cases, generate anxiety, difficulty concentrating, or energy fatigue. To help the child deal with these demands, the Arcturians suggest integrating practices such as crystal therapy, aromatherapy, and therapeutic play, which act simultaneously on the physical, emotional, and energetic bodies.

Crystal therapy, in this context, can be applied as follows:

Choose suitable crystals, such as clear quartz (mental clarity), fluorite (concentration), and black tourmaline (energetic protection).

Before the start of school activities, the child can hold a small crystal for a few minutes, breathing deeply.

At home, after returning from school, a small ritual of energy cleansing can be created, placing the crystals on the child's body (main chakras) for about 10 minutes, with the intention of releasing accumulated tensions.

Aromatherapy can be incorporated into the routine with the use of environmental diffusers, especially during study and rest times. Essential oils such as lavender (relaxation), sweet orange (joy), and rosemary (focus) can be used according to the need of the moment, always in dilutions suitable for children.

Therapeutic play, in turn, offers a safe space for the child to express their emotions, elaborate internal conflicts, and strengthen emotional bonds. Stories created together, pretend play, and storytelling with magical and symbolic elements are ways to allow the child to interact playfully with their emotions and subtle perceptions, without the rigidity of rational words.

In all these phases, connection with nature remains a central axis of care and promotion of integral health. Every outdoor walk, every touch of the earth or encounter with an animal, every observation of the moon and stars are recognized as experiences that reactivate the child's cosmic memory, helping them to feel part of something bigger, where their physical body, their soul, and the Earth itself dance in harmony. This spontaneous dialogue with nature nourishes the immune system, strengthens creativity, and teaches, in an organic way, about cycles, impermanence, and the interconnection of all forms of life.

Finally, attentive listening and respect for the uniqueness of each child are sacred values within the Arcturian perspective. Each being that comes into the world carries a unique combination of gifts, memories, and purposes, and it is up to the adults around them to become guardians of this journey, offering clear but loving boundaries, while cultivating empathetic listening, validation of emotions, and encouragement of creativity. In this space of love and respect, each child blossoms like an incarnated star, capable of radiating their unique light and, at the same time, recognizing themselves as part of the great cosmos in eternal expansion.

In this continuous and loving care, child health is revealed as a process of co-creation between the child, their family, nature, and the subtle flows of the universe, where every attentive look, every welcoming gesture, and every space of freedom and belonging nourishes not only the body and mind, but also the soul in its earthly awakening. By recognizing the child as a living bridge between the spiritual world and matter, the Arcturians invite us to honor their innate sensitivity and silent wisdom, allowing them to grow with the confidence that they are safe to be who they came to be. Thus, childhood, lived with respect for the essence and time of each being, is transformed not only into a phase of growth but into a sacred soul walk, where health, love, and purpose dance intertwined, guiding each step of the journey.

Chapter 21
The Importance of Mindful Eating

Mindful eating represents a profound path of reconnection between the human being, nature, and the essential energy that permeates all forms of life. Each food carries not only a biochemical composition of nutrients but also a unique vibrational signature, resulting from its origin, cultivation, handling, and the intention present in all stages of its production. By understanding that the act of eating goes beyond the mechanical ingestion of calories and vitamins, it becomes possible to perceive that mindful nutrition is, above all, an invitation to presence, reverence, and the intentional choice of each element that makes up the daily diet. More than satisfying a physiological need, eating mindfully is integrating the ancestral wisdom of food and its subtle properties, respecting its natural cycle, its vital energy, and its role in sustaining bodily and spiritual harmony. This approach is anchored in the perception that each meal is an opportunity to align body, mind, and spirit, transforming the simple act of eating into a sacred ritual of connection with the forces of nature and the cosmic flows that sustain life in its entirety.

In the context of Arcturian wisdom, mindful eating transcends the dichotomy between healthy and unhealthy, expanding the understanding to the vibrational frequency of food and its ability to directly influence consciousness and energy fields. The Arcturians recognize that each food has an energy matrix that resonates with specific patterns of the human vibrational field, and can strengthen or destabilize the flow of vital energy that circulates in the body. Fruits harvested at their right time, vegetables grown with respect and care, seeds preserved in their original purity, and minimally processed foods carry an intact energetic memory, capable of harmonizing the subtle bodies and promoting states of physical, emotional, and spiritual balance. This understanding reflects the holistic view that each food choice is not isolated but part of an interdependent process between individual, environment, and cosmos. Thus, the act of eating mindfully implies recognizing food as an extension of the Earth's own energy, as a vehicle for cosmic information, and as an opportunity to align oneself with the highest vibrations of creation, actively participating in the maintenance of planetary and personal balance.

Cultivating food awareness, in this sense, involves not only the careful selection of ingredients but also the posture of reverence and gratitude that permeates the entire process of preparation and consumption. Each stage – from the choice of food, through the act of cooking with loving intention, to the practice of eating with full attention – constitutes an opportunity to nourish not only the physical body but also the subtle energy that sustains integral vitality. Conscious presence during meals, the sharpened perception of flavors, textures, and aromas, and attentive listening to the body's signals allow us to recover the innate wisdom of recognizing what truly nourishes and strengthens. This state of presence transforms the relationship with food into a sensitive dialogue, where each meal becomes a ceremony of integration between body, soul, and universe. Thus, mindful eating establishes itself as a fundamental pillar for strengthening integral health and expanding consciousness, providing not only physical and emotional balance but also the subtle vibrational elevation necessary for the flourishing of an existence aligned with natural and universal laws.

The influence of food on physical and energetic health is revealed in deep and interconnected layers, starting from the essential understanding that each food is a unique source of vital energy and nutrients indispensable for the harmonious functioning of body and mind. It is not just about ingesting calories or balancing macronutrients mechanically, but about recognizing that the subtle vibration present in each food dialogues directly with the human energy fields. When this connection is neglected and the diet becomes dominated by ultra-processed, refined products full of chemical additives, blockages in the natural flow of vital energy are established. These artificial substances, when introduced into the body, create zones of energetic densification, capable of generating silent inflammations, hormonal imbalances, and distortions in the vibrational patterns that sustain physical and emotional balance. In contrast, the conscious choice of whole foods, of organic origin and rich in living nutrients, not only nourishes the physical body efficiently but also elevates personal vibration, expanding perception and strengthening the subtle energy field.

This distinction between foods that drain or restore vitality is deeply supported by the Arcturian approach, which understands food as a vehicle of cosmic energy condensed into matter. Vibrational foods, such as fresh fruits, vegetables harvested at the right time, greens that sprouted in nourished and respected soil, whole grains free of genetic manipulation, seeds loaded with germination power, and oilseeds preserved in their original purity, act as true energetic modulators. Each of these foods carries in its structure the vibrational memory of the Earth and the informational code of sunlight, functioning as messengers of vitality and harmony for the physical and subtle bodies. Eating these foods with awareness, therefore, is opening space for the organism itself to tune in to higher frequencies, dissolving dense patterns and restoring the free flow of vital energy.

Foods that promote healing and balance, from the Arcturian perspective, are not only those rich in biochemical nutrients but mainly those that preserve the vibrational integrity of their origin. They are foods that arrive at the table close to their natural state, harvested and cultivated in cycles that respect the rhythms of nature, free of pesticides, herbicides, preservatives, and artificial additives that corrupt their original energy matrix. The choice of fresh, seasonal, locally produced, and small-scale foods favors not only the maintenance of their nutrients in an integral state but also preserves the pulsating vital energy, essential to promote balance and healing. Diversity in food is equally valued, not only to guarantee a wide range of vitamins, minerals, and bioactive compounds but also to stimulate the senses and nourish the soul with the beauty and the chromatic and sensory intelligence of food.

In this sense, the practice of combining foods of different colors, flavors, and textures is a subtle and powerful way to align the physical and energetic bodies. Each color carries a specific vibrational frequency, resonating with different energy centers of the body. Red foods, for example, strengthen the vitality and energy of action associated with the root chakra; green foods nourish the heart center, expanding the capacity for compassion and connection; and violet or bluish foods fine-tune intuitive perception, favoring mental clarity. In this way, the colorful plate becomes a healing mandala, a vibrational composition that acts simultaneously on cellular nutrition and the harmonization of the subtle bodies.

Alongside the careful choice of food, the practice of moderation emerges as a fundamental pillar to preserve internal harmony. Overeating, even healthy foods, overloads energy flows and obscures subtle perception. Moderation, combined with attentive listening to the internal signals of hunger and satiety, allows the body to determine its real needs, adjusting the volume and rhythm of meals to its capacity for assimilation. This sensitive practice of self-regulation is reinforced by the Arcturian guidance to trust intuition to guide food choices. More than following rigid diets or fixed rules, learning to decode the subtle signals of one's own body is an invitation to profound self-knowledge and the construction of a loving and respectful relationship with the act of nourishing oneself.

The preparation of food, in turn, is elevated to the condition of a sacred act, where the energy of the cook is transferred to the food through the loving intention that permeates each gesture. The Arcturians teach that the energy of those who handle the ingredients, the clarity of intention, and the emotional vibration present during preparation are as important as the intrinsic quality of the food itself. Cooking in a state of presence, infusing gratitude and love into each cut, each mixture, and each cooking process, creates a favorable energy matrix that amplifies the therapeutic effects of food.

Creating a calm and welcoming environment for meals is equally essential to nourish not only the physical body but also the subtle field. A harmonious space, free from distractions and imbued with serenity, favors full attention to the act of eating and receptivity to the subtle information present in each food. This environment can be enriched with small rituals of gratitude, such as lighting a candle or silently expressing recognition for the journey that each food has taken to reach the table. This reverent connection expands the awareness of interdependence and rescues the inherent sacredness of the act of eating.

The practice of slow and conscious chewing is another essential key within the Arcturian approach. Chewing each food with full attention not only facilitates the digestive process, allowing enzymes to work effectively, but also tunes consciousness to the subtle vibrational messages contained in each bite. This slow pace favors the full perception of flavors, aromas, and textures, awakening the senses and expanding satisfaction, reducing compulsion, and strengthening the intuitive connection with one's own body.

To guide this practice, a simple and powerful technique can be adopted:
1. Before starting the meal, take a few deep breaths, connecting with the present moment.
2. Observe the appearance of the food, its colors, shapes, and textures.
3. With each bite, chew slowly, trying to identify layers of flavor and textural sensations.
4. Avoid distractions, such as electronic devices, to maintain full attention on the act of eating.
5. At the end of the meal, dedicate a brief moment to give thanks, recognizing the elements of nature and all the beings involved in the production of that food.

Expressing gratitude for the food received is more than a symbolic gesture; it is a vibrational alignment that strengthens the link between individual, nature, and cosmos. This practice of gratitude does not need to follow rigid formulas. It can be a simple silent nod of the head, a thought of recognition, or a brief prayer that springs spontaneously from the heart. The important thing is that gratitude is accompanied by the awareness that each food is a gift from the Earth, a gift that sustains the continuity of life and nourishes the evolutionary path of each being.

In this way, mindful and loving eating, practiced with presence, respect, and reverence, transcends physical nutrition and becomes a powerful tool for healing and vibrational elevation. Each meal, then, is lived as a sacred opportunity to align body, mind, and spirit, actively participating in the creation of a more harmonious and luminous reality, where the simple act of eating becomes a celebration of existence itself.

In this harmonious flow between food, body, and consciousness, mindful eating ceases to be just a care for health and transforms into a subtle and continuous dialogue between the being and the universe. Every choice, every preparation, and every meal become portals of self-knowledge and reconnection, where nutrition goes far beyond sustaining matter—it strengthens the loving bond with the Earth, fine-tunes inner listening, and aligns the subtle fields with the greater intelligence of life. Eating, then, becomes a gesture of belonging and reverence, a daily reminder that each being is both the one who harvests and the one who is nourished, and that in this sacred cycle of giving and receiving lies the essence of universal harmony.

Chapter 22
Physical Exercises and Movement

From the Arcturian perspective, body movement is understood as a natural expression of vital energy in constant flux, a continuous dialogue between the physical body and the subtle fields of consciousness that permeate it. Every gesture, every stretch, every movement of the body is not just an isolated biomechanical action, but a reflection of the harmony or disharmony existing between the mind, emotions, and vital energy. For the Arcturians, the human body was not designed for prolonged inertia, but rather to be a channel for the fluid expression of cosmic life force, capable of absorbing, circulating, and releasing energies in continuous motion. Thus, the practice of physical exercises and conscious movements becomes a fundamental mechanism to preserve the harmonic flow of energy in the meridians and chakras, prevent blockages that result in illness, and, above all, expand body awareness as an indivisible part of higher consciousness. Every conscious movement, no matter how simple, opens portals of connection between the physical and the subtle, allowing the practitioner not only to condition their body but also to tune their personal vibration with the harmonious pulsation of the universe.

By incorporating movement into the daily routine under this expanded perspective, each exercise ceases to be an effort aimed only at physical conditioning and becomes a meditative act in itself, a ritual of full presence and attentive listening to the messages of one's own body. The Arcturians teach that the human body is a living library, full of ancestral records and information about energy patterns accumulated throughout life and previous existences. Conscious movement, performed with intention and attention, allows access to these records, dissolving crystallized tensions and realigning the energy structure in a smooth and continuous way. Walking in the midst of nature, for example, ceases to be a simple physical activity and becomes an invitation to energetic fusion with the intelligence of the Earth, allowing each step to resonate like a beat in tune with the planetary heart. Likewise, practices such as yoga, tai chi, and intuitive dances are understood as languages of the spiritualized body, capable of integrating emotion, mind, and spirit in a single harmonious flow of creative expression.

In addition to its energetic and healing functions, conscious movement plays an essential role in strengthening the bond between the individual and their physical vehicle, restoring the perception of the body as a sacred temple that houses consciousness and serves as a bridge to earthly experience. Each mobilized joint, each stretched muscle, each breath synchronized with the body gesture becomes an act of reverence and loving care, expanding body awareness and strengthening the sense of belonging to one's own body. This renewed connection with the physical body rescues the instinctive wisdom of recognizing one's own limits and needs, avoiding excesses and allowing the practice of movement to be adjusted in tune with the present moment of each being. Thus, by respecting body intelligence and flowing with its natural needs and rhythms, conscious movement is consolidated as a fundamental pillar of self-healing, expansion of consciousness, and full integration of the being, promoting integral health and vibrational alignment with the harmonious flows of cosmic existence.

The importance of movement in physical and energetic health lies, first of all, in the deep understanding that the human body is not a static structure, but a dynamic composition of tissues, fluids, energy, and consciousness in constant interaction. The body was designed to move, to explore different ranges of motion, to adapt to the environment, and, through this adaptation, to expand its capabilities of perception and response. Every cell, every muscle, and every joint carries within it the memory of movement, from the first moments of intrauterine life to the most complex gestures developed throughout existence. It is through movement that blood circulates more efficiently, transporting oxygen and nutrients to all parts of the organism, revitalizing tissues, and promoting cell regeneration. At the same time, movement actively contributes to the elimination of toxins, both through the activation of the lymphatic system and the release of substances accumulated in the muscles and organs, allowing the body to maintain its chemical and energetic balance.

This dynamic, however, goes beyond physiology. By moving with awareness, each human being has the opportunity to release not only physical toxins but also dense energies that accumulate over time. Emotional tensions, repressed memories, and energy blockages can be gently dissolved when movement is guided by an intention of cleansing and harmonization. The chakras, centers of vital energy, are directly impacted by the quality of movement, being able to expand and flow freely when the body expresses itself in a fluid and harmonious way. Through the consistent practice of physical exercises, not only is the physical structure strengthened — muscles, bones, tendons, and joints — but also a kind of vibrational pathway is created through which vital energy can circulate more easily. This continuous flow of vital energy, known by so many names in different traditions, is the basis of the feeling of genuine well-being, that silent peace that arises when body, mind, and spirit dance in perfect harmony.

Among the most recommended practices within this expanded Arcturian perspective, those that combine fluid movement and conscious presence stand out. Regular walks, especially in the midst of nature, become much more than cardiovascular exercise. Each step can be transformed into a gesture of connection with the pulsation of the Earth, allowing the telluric energy to rise through the soles of the feet and nourish the lower energy centers. Walking, then, ceases to be a simple physical activity and becomes a ritual of integration between the being and the planet. Similarly, practices such as yoga and tai chi chuan offer precious opportunities to cultivate flexibility, not only physical but also mental and emotional. Each sustained posture in yoga or each fluid sequence of tai chi is a meditation in motion, where the breath guides the rhythm and the body learns to align itself with the subtle flows of energy that permeate it.

Dance, especially in its spontaneous and intuitive form, is another essential practice in this context. When the body is invited to move freely, without pre-defined choreography or external judgments, it becomes an instrument of direct expression of the soul. Music, or even silence, serves as a backdrop for the body to draw its emotions, its stories, and its non-verbal prayers in space. In this process, not only is motor coordination, cardiovascular endurance, or flexibility worked, but crystallized emotions are also released, allowing vital energy to recover its natural flow.

For those seeking a more structured approach, adapted to their specific needs, it is possible to create personalized routines that integrate gentle stretching, progressive muscle strengthening, and balance and coordination exercises. The secret is to adjust the practice to the present moment of each body, respecting its limitations and celebrating its capabilities, without comparisons or excessive demands. Instead of following rigid patterns, the practice becomes a continuous dialogue between body and consciousness, where each exercise is an opportunity for self-knowledge and self-care.

Practicing outdoors, whenever possible, adds another layer of benefit to this approach. Being in contact with the elements of nature — feeling the wind on the skin, the texture of the earth under the feet, the heat of the sun, or the humidity of the air — expands sensory and energetic perception. Each movement performed in this context is potentiated by the constant exchange of energy with the environment, creating a synergy between the physical body and the planetary body. The soil, the air, the water, and the light become allies in the process of revitalization and healing.

Regarding the integration between movement, meditation, and energy healing, there are specific techniques that can be incorporated gradually, as the practitioner develops greater sensitivity and body awareness. One of these techniques consists of starting each movement session with a brief pause for internalization, where attention is directed to the breath and the perception of one's own body. Feeling the contact of the feet with the ground, perceiving the flow of the breath, and recognizing areas of tension or discomfort prepares the ground for the following movement to be guided by attentive listening.

With consciousness anchored in the present moment, each movement can then be synchronized with the breath. On the inhale, visualize vital energy entering through the top of the head or the soles of the feet, filling the body with light and vitality. On the exhale, visualize the release of tensions, dense emotions, or energy blockages, allowing the body to become lighter and more fluid. This simple practice of coordination between movement and breathing transforms any sequence of stretches or everyday gestures into a true energy practice.

Another complementary technique involves creative visualization. While the body moves, whether in a walk, in a series of yoga postures, or in a spontaneous dance, the practitioner is invited to imagine energy flowing freely through their energy system. One can visualize the golden energy of life force running through the spine, or a soft blue light enveloping the joints and dissolving any stiffness. This directed visualization enhances the therapeutic effects of movement, creating a bridge between the physical body and the subtle bodies.

As a fundamental part of this integration process, the practice of gratitude for the moving body deserves to be highlighted. At the end of each practice, or even during the most challenging movements, taking a moment to thank one's own body for its ability to move, adapt, and express itself reinforces the loving connection between consciousness and the physical vehicle. This simple gesture of gratitude, when repeated regularly, transforms body practice into a celebration of embodied life, dissolving the fragmented view that separates body, mind, and spirit.

Thus, by adopting an expanded perspective on movement, where each gesture is recognized as an extension of consciousness and each physical practice is understood as a ritual of integration, the human being begins to perceive their own body as a sacred ally on the path of healing and expansion of consciousness. In this way, movement ceases to be an obligation or a mere instrument of physical conditioning and becomes a living portal of connection with the essence, a subtle vehicle of communication with the cosmos, and a silent language of reverence for one's own existence.

In this continuous flow between body and consciousness, each conscious movement becomes a gesture of alignment with the greater purpose of the incarnated soul, dissolving the old separation between the physical and the spiritual. The body, honored as a living field of expression of universal energy, reveals itself not only as a vehicle of experiences but as a sensitive mirror of the inner journey, reflecting in gestures, postures, and rhythms the unique history of each being. Thus, the act of moving becomes an active and loving listening, where the body itself whispers its memories, desires, and forgotten wisdoms, inviting the human being to dance in harmony with the cycles of life, integrating presence, fluidity, and reverence in each step of their earthly journey.

Chapter 23
The Power of Restorative Sleep

Restorative sleep is an essential portal of multidimensional regeneration, in which the physical body, the mind, and the subtle bodies enter a synchronized state of restoration and energetic realignment. Far beyond the simple suspension of wakefulness, sleep is understood as a sacred cycle, in which the organism not only recovers its physical vitality through biochemical and cellular processes but also participates in a broader flow of integration between planes of existence. During this period, consciousness shifts beyond ordinary sensory perceptions and accesses subtle levels of learning, healing, and spiritual connection. With each cycle of deep sleep, the energy field is recalibrated, information gathered throughout the day is processed and adjusted, and channels of communication with higher dimensions open for exchanges of knowledge and spiritual guidance. This understanding expands the notion of rest, repositioning sleep as a dynamic process of vibrational alignment, where integral health is co-created between the physical body and the spiritual spheres that sustain it.

In the Arcturian view, each stage of sleep is an opportunity to rebalance not only the physiological systems but also the vital energy flows that run through the meridians, chakras, and subtle bodies. During deep sleep, there is an intense energetic purification, in which blockages, emotional residues, and accumulated tensions are dissolved or softened, allowing the vital energy to flow more freely upon awakening. This process of energetic detoxification is essential to maintain vibrational harmony, preventing subtle imbalances from crystallizing in the physical body as symptoms or diseases. Furthermore, sleep is seen as a period in which the soul, freed from the constraints of linear perception, accesses chambers of healing and learning in higher planes. In these spaces, consciousness is nourished by harmonic frequencies, receives insights for personal challenges, and participates in evolutionary exchanges with beings of light and spiritual masters, who assist in the process of expanding consciousness and updating the energy codes necessary for the next waking cycle.

For sleep to fully play its regenerative and evolutionary role, it is necessary to create material and subtle conditions that favor this deep immersion. The physical environment, the mental and emotional state before sleep, and the conscious intention to open oneself to regeneration and spiritual connection are fundamental components of this preparation. An organized, clean, and energetically harmonized room, free of electromagnetic pollution and excessive visual stimuli, functions as a vibrational sanctuary that welcomes and protects the body and soul during rest. The choice of natural bedding, with soft textures, and the presence of elements that radiate high frequencies, such as crystals and purifying plants, contribute to creating a vibrational field conducive to deep and restorative sleep. Likewise, transition rituals between wakefulness and sleep, such as relaxing baths, guided meditations, and conscious breathing practices, help to slow down the mind and prepare the energy field to cross the threshold between worlds with serenity and receptivity. Thus, restorative sleep reveals itself not only as a vital physiological function but as a sacred link between earthly experience and the spiritual realms, sustaining integral balance and promoting the evolution of consciousness at all levels of being.

From the Arcturian perspective, sleep is not just the suspension of wakefulness or the shutting down of the physical body for simple rest. It is understood as an expanded state of consciousness, where the physical body retreats into its self-repair processes, while the astral body frees itself from the dense bonds of matter and projects itself into more subtle dimensions. This dual journey, simultaneous and complementary, is what guarantees not only cellular and physiological renewal but also energetic, emotional, and spiritual renewal. While the physical body, silent in its bed, performs its meticulous tasks of cell repair, tissue regeneration, biochemical reorganization, and deep detoxification of the systems, the astral body, lighter and more fluid, crosses the vibrational portals that open when the conscious mind falls asleep. It is through this dimensional freedom that the astral body dives into parallel realities, meets with beings of light, travels through temples of healing and learning, and receives instructions and codifications that nourish the evolution of the incarnated consciousness.

The quality of this sleep, that is, the depth with which the physical body surrenders and the clarity with which the astral body moves to these subtle spheres, has direct and profound reflections on all aspects of human health. Truly restorative sleep is capable of strengthening the immune system, restoring organic vitality from the subtlest layers of the energy matrix. It also harmonizes emotional flows, dissolving tensions accumulated during the day and reframing experiences that, otherwise, would crystallize dissonant patterns in the energy field. The mind awakens from this immersion clearer and more lucid, as if the veils of everyday confusion were loosened by the combined action of physical repair and spiritual nourishment. Consciousness, by being bathed in these higher frequencies, expands beyond the limits of the immediate identity, recognizing itself as part of a larger flow of cosmic intelligence and love. The result is a more centered, vital, and aligned state of being, where body, mind, and soul dance in harmony with the natural rhythms of the universe.

For this sleep to fully fulfill its restorative and evolutionary role, the Arcturian tradition suggests not only an attitude of surrender and respect for rest, but a series of techniques and practices that prepare the body, the environment, and the energy field for this crossing.

Creating a conducive environment is one of the first steps and involves not only the physical arrangement of the space, but its subtle vibrational harmonization. The room should be organized with care, free of excesses and unnecessary objects that can create energetic turbulence. Each object present should have a reason for being and radiate harmony, functioning as a silent guardian of this sanctuary of rest. The physical and energetic cleansing of the space is fundamental, and regular smudging with herbs such as lavender, rosemary, or white sage is recommended, which purify the environment and elevate its frequency.

Darkness is also a precious element in this context, as the absence of artificial light stimuli favors the natural regulation of melatonin production, the hormone that signals to the body the time to retreat and regenerate. Avoiding intense lights in the hours before sleep and preferring softer, yellowish sources of illumination creates a smooth transition between wakefulness and rest. If necessary, blackout curtains can be used to block external lights, creating a protective cocoon that favors deep immersion in the layers of restorative sleep.

In addition to the physical space, the preparation of the body and mind for sleep is treated with reverence. The practice of relaxing rituals before sleep signals to the nervous system that it is safe to slow down and surrender to rest. Among these rituals, warm baths are particularly valued. Immersion in warm water, especially when enriched with magnesium salts or calming essential oils such as lavender or chamomile, helps to release muscle tension and dissolve electromagnetic charges accumulated throughout the day. Water, in its ancestral intelligence, not only cleanses the physical body but reconnects the being to its natural fluidity, paving the way for deeper and more restorative sleep.

Reading inspiring texts or listening to soft music are also recommended practices, provided they choose content that inspires calm, beauty, and spiritual connection. Avoiding dense or excessively stimulating information preserves the mental field from unnecessary agitation, allowing it to surrender more easily to the flow of sleep. Similarly, the practice of conscious breathing is an invitation for body and mind to enter into resonance, synchronizing internal rhythms with the subtle flows of the universe. Breathing deeply, in a rhythmic and attentive way, activates the parasympathetic system, which signals to the organism that it is time for retreat and regeneration.

The use of crystals is another precious resource within the Arcturian approach to restorative sleep. Crystals such as amethyst, known for its ability to raise the frequency of the environment and facilitate spiritual contact, can be positioned next to the bed or under the pillow. Rose quartz, with its loving and welcoming vibration, helps to dissolve emotional tensions, creating a field of serenity conducive to surrender. Crystals should be periodically cleaned and programmed to maintain their function as guardians of sacred sleep.

Essential oils, with their therapeutic and vibrational properties, also play a fundamental role.

Diffusers can spread, throughout the room, the subtle essence of lavender, cedarwood, or chamomile, creating an atmosphere of welcome and protection. Applying a few drops directly to the wrists or soles of the feet before sleep works as a sign of affection and care for the body, inviting it to relax deeply.

Visualization and meditation techniques before sleep are, perhaps, one of the most valued practices in the Arcturian perspective. Lying in a comfortable position, gently closing the eyes, and visualizing a sphere of golden light enveloping the entire body is a simple and powerful way to align with higher frequencies. This sphere can be imagined as a protective cocoon, within which the physical body is restored and the astral body prepares for its nocturnal journey. One breathes within this sphere, perceiving it pulsating in tune with the heartbeat, until the conscious mind dissolves in the tranquil flow of sleep.

The so-called sleep hygiene is an integral part of this approach and involves adjustments to daytime habits that directly reflect on the quality of nighttime rest. Creating a regular routine of times to sleep and wake up, avoiding abrupt variations, teaches the body to enter into resonance with natural cycles. Avoiding caffeine and alcohol in the hours before sleep preserves the delicate brain chemistry that sustains natural sleep. Likewise, the practice of physical activities during the day, especially in contact with nature, harmonizes circadian rhythms, grounding the body in its primordial wisdom.

In this way, restorative sleep, seen through the Arcturian prism, is much more than a physiological function. It is a portal of healing, reconnection, and evolution. Each night well slept is a sacred opportunity for body and soul to realign with the divine essence, restoring not only physical vitality but spiritual clarity and the purpose of existence. Sleeping thus becomes an act of deep reverence for one's own journey, a moment where the veils between the worlds thin and the soul, free and full, breathes the cosmic breath that sustains it.

And it is in this silent immersion, where the breath of the body intertwines with the rhythms of the cosmos, that restorative sleep reveals its true essence: a return to the inner home, where the being sheds the layers accumulated during the day and rediscovers the softness of its own light. Each night lived with this awareness transforms rest into a sacred altar of healing and reunion, where the body is honored, the soul is nourished, and consciousness is elevated. Sleeping, then, ceases to be just a physiological necessity and becomes an act of full trust in the intelligence of life, a cycle of surrender and rebirth that sustains, night after night, the blossoming of the being in its journey between worlds.

Chapter 24
The Healing of the Soul and Life Purpose

The healing of the soul represents a profound journey of reconnection with the purest essence of being, where every experience lived, every pain faced, and every lesson assimilated converge to reveal the greater purpose that guides existence. In this path of self-discovery, it is understood that the soul is not just an isolated spark in search of growth, but rather a singular expression of a larger cosmic consciousness, intertwined with the universal web of life. Emotional wounds, ancestral traumas, and inherited conditioning, both from this and other incarnations, form subtle layers that obscure this original essence, hindering the authentic expression of life purpose. The healing of the soul, therefore, is not limited to the release of pain and repressed memories, but expands to the rescue of innate wisdom, inner truth, and the sacred alliance between the individual soul and the collective purpose of existence. Each stage of this healing journey offers the opportunity to transmute accumulated densities into integrated lessons, allowing the soul to regain its clarity, brilliance, and alignment with the natural flow of creation.

In the Arcturian view, the healing of the soul is inseparable from the manifestation of life purpose, because it is precisely in the process of recognizing and integrating the fragmented parts of consciousness that the true path of being is revealed. Every challenge overcome, every limiting belief dissolved, and every ancestral pattern transmuted releases layers of crystallized energy that prevented the soul from radiating its unique signature in the world. From this state of clarity and reintegration, the connection with life purpose emerges not as an external goal to be pursued, but as an inevitable inner calling, an essential vibration that resonates from the center of being. Discovering and manifesting this purpose is an act of profound alignment between the personal essence and the creative flow of the universe, where talents, passions, and natural gifts become spontaneous expressions of the soul in service to collective evolution. Arcturian medicine understands that, by healing and recognizing their purpose, each human being contributes directly to the elevation of planetary consciousness, as each soul aligned with its essential truth becomes a source of inspiration, healing, and expansion for everyone around them.

This journey of healing and self-discovery, however, requires commitment, humility, and a willingness to look deeply into the inner shadows, welcoming them with compassion and transforming them into practical wisdom. Constant self-observation allows one to recognize the automatic patterns that perpetuate suffering, while the loving acceptance of emotions interrupts cycles of repression and denial, opening space for genuine healing. Practices such as meditation, conscious breathing, and creative visualization are powerful allies to access the deepest records of the soul and dissolve energetic blockages that limit the full expression of being. Alongside these practices, gratitude and forgiveness emerge as master keys to the healing of the soul, as they elevate personal vibration, reframe lived experiences, and free consciousness from the shackles of the past. Thus, the healing of the soul and the discovery of life purpose become a single ascending path of return to the inner home, where the being recognizes its divine essence and fully expresses its light, fulfilling the unique role that only it can play in the great plan of creation.

Arcturian medicine, when entering the intricacies of soul healing, promotes a deep process of reintegration of fragmented parts of consciousness, allowing aspects that were once denied or dispersed to reoccupy their natural space in the totality of being. Each rescued fragment represents a memory, a trace of identity, or an ancestral skill that, for various reasons, was dissociated from the main consciousness. Throughout countless life experiences, whether in this incarnation or in past journeys, the soul has often faced traumatic situations or challenges that, because they were not understood or processed, were encapsulated in pockets of dense energy. These pockets, like small grains of sand in the crystalline flow of consciousness, generate perceptual distortions, repetitive behavior patterns, and pain that seem to have no logical explanation. It is in this subtle terrain that Arcturian medicine acts, using a combination of vibrational techniques and spiritual technologies to dissolve these layers and restore the original harmony.

The journey of soul healing inevitably passes through the exploration of past lives, a dive into the Akashic records where all the experiences of the soul throughout its evolutionary trajectory are stored. It is not just about revisiting these events as if flipping through the pages of an old book, but about allowing the emotional, energetic, and symbolic content of these memories to come to the surface to be understood, welcomed, and transmuted. In many cases, soul contracts signed in other existences — conscious or unconscious agreements made with other beings or even with spiritual groups — continue to reverberate as invisible chains that influence choices and block the full expression of being. Arcturian medicine assists in the identification and revision of these contracts, allowing the being to assess whether they still serve their growth or if, on the contrary, they have become invisible prisons that limit the flow of the soul. In this process, conscious free will is restored, allowing the soul to free itself from old pacts and reintegrate sovereignty over its own destiny.

The release of karmas is another essential facet of this process. Karma, understood not as punishment, but as learning in action, is revisited and reframed in the light of the expanded understanding that arises when the soul accesses its innate wisdom. Each karmic situation, each challenging encounter or repetition of painful patterns, reveals itself as an invitation to healing and integration. Instead of being an endless cycle of cause and effect, karma transforms into a compassionate teacher that points to the areas where love and acceptance have not yet fully blossomed. By dissolving these karmic layers and integrating the lessons learned, the soul is freed to express its authenticity, without the invisible shackles of the past.

Within this approach, Arcturian medicine is anchored in a series of subtle and powerful techniques, each of them adapted to the specific need of the soul in its current stage of evolution. Meditation, for example, is not just a moment of silence and introspection, but a vibrational recalibration tool that allows the higher consciousness of the soul to override the noise of the conditioned mind. Through creative visualization, the soul is guided to reconstruct internal landscapes, reframe traumatic memories, and anchor symbolic images of healing that reverberate directly in the emotional and energetic body.

The reprogramming of spiritual DNA is another fundamental practice. Through the conscious activation of light codes stored in the multidimensional layers of DNA, inherited patterns of pain, limitation, and disconnection can be dissolved, giving way to the full expression of the soul's unique gifts and potentials. This reprogramming occurs both vibrationally, through sound intonations and sacred geometries, and consciously, through affirmations and decrees that anchor new realities in the quantum field of being.

Past life therapy complements this set, functioning as a bridge between the present and the ancestral memories that still echo in the psyche.

Through an expanded state of consciousness, the soul revisits key moments of its journey, not only to observe, but to actively interact with these memories, offering itself the acceptance, understanding, and release that were not possible at the original moment. This temporal reintegration dissolves blockages and rescues talents and wisdom that were frozen in other timelines.

Another essential pillar of Arcturian medicine is the channeling of information. In this context, the soul receives directly from its higher essence — or from related spiritual guides — insights and specific guidance for its process of healing and realignment. These messages, sometimes symbolic and sometimes extremely direct, function as internal maps that illuminate the next step on the soul's journey.

To sustain this process of healing and reintegration, some daily practices become indispensable. Constant self-observation is one of them, as it allows the identification of emotional triggers, recurring thoughts, and behaviors that perpetuate cycles of pain. By recognizing these patterns with lucidity and without judgment, the soul begins the process of disengaging from these automatic programs. At the same time, the loving acceptance of all emotions — without censorship or repression — allows the natural energy flow to be restored, dissolving emotional knots accumulated over time.

The healthy expression of feelings is equally fundamental. Communicating one's own needs authentically, establishing clear and respectful boundaries, and sharing vulnerabilities without fear are practices that strengthen relationships and create an environment where the soul's truth can flourish. Alongside this, the reprogramming of limiting beliefs is worked on systematically, replacing internal narratives of incapacity, guilt, or unworthiness with affirmations of power, deservingness, and divine connection.

Forgiveness, as a conscious practice, reveals itself as a master key to the healing of the soul. It does not mean forgetting or justifying, but releasing the emotional weight that anchors the soul in the past. By forgiving — both oneself and others — the soul dissolves the invisible chains of resentment and reopens the flow of unconditional love, allowing inner peace to occupy the space previously filled by hurts and guilt.

And, finally, gratitude becomes the fundamental frequency that anchors and expands all this healing. By recognizing the blessings already received, by thanking for the lessons learned — even the most challenging ones — and by celebrating every small victory on the path of reintegration, the soul elevates its vibration and strengthens its connection with the divine. Gratitude transforms the gaze, allowing the soul to perceive the beauty and purpose in every detail of existence, reframing scars as sacred marks of a unique journey.

In this continuous spiral of healing and self-discovery, Arcturian medicine does not present itself as an external solution or a rigid protocol, but as a loving invitation to the soul to become its own healer, rediscovering within itself the keys to its fullness and aligning itself, step by step, with the greater purpose that called it into existence.

And it is in this conscious return to the center of one's own soul that true healing is revealed: not as an end point or a promise of perfection, but as a living movement of remembering who one is, of honoring each integrated fragment, and of expressing, with courage and delicacy, the uniqueness of one's own light. Life purpose, far from being a distant goal, emerges as the inner voice that has always been there, whispering between the pains and silences, awaiting the moment when the soul, free from the shackles of fear and forgetfulness, finally recognizes itself as an essential part of the great cosmic mosaic. And so, the healing of the soul and the manifestation of purpose become faces of the same awakening: the intimate dance between being and existence, where each step is sacred and each expression of inner truth illuminates not only one's own path, but also that of all those who walk around.

Chapter 25
Integration with Conventional Medicine

The integration of Arcturian medicine and conventional medicine represents a crucial advancement in the expanded understanding of health, bringing together the scientific rigor of Western medicine with the vibrational and energetic depth of Arcturian wisdom. This fusion does not imply the replacement of one approach by the other, but the creation of a space for cooperation and synergy, where each perspective complements and enhances the other. Conventional medicine, with its evidence-based methods, provides precise diagnoses and essential interventions in acute, emergency, and surgical situations. In parallel, Arcturian medicine expands the view beyond the physical symptom, delving into the energetic and spiritual matrix that sustains and influences the manifestation of diseases, identifying imbalances in the subtle field, ancestral traumas, or misaligned vibrational patterns that contribute to the weakening of the physical body. Together, these approaches form a comprehensive model of care, capable of contemplating the human being as an integrated system of body, mind, emotions, and soul, whose full health depends on the harmony between these levels.

This integration happens most effectively when doctors, energy therapists, and patients adopt a posture of open dialogue and mutual respect, recognizing that each approach has its strengths and limitations. Conventional medicine, by using laboratory tests, imaging techniques, and scientifically validated therapeutic protocols, provides a clear mapping of the patient's physical state and the biological processes in progress. Arcturian medicine, in turn, uses vibrational reading tools, channeling of information from the morphogenetic field, and energetic harmonization techniques to access the invisible dimension of health, offering a broader understanding of the origins of dysfunctions and pointing out paths of healing that involve reprogramming beliefs, releasing traumatic memories, and reconnecting with the spiritual essence. This dialogue between knowledge allows the construction of individualized therapeutic plans, where conventional treatments can be enhanced by vibrational and spiritual practices, strengthening not only the physical body but also the emotional resilience and mental clarity of the patient throughout the healing process.

The successful integration of these approaches requires not only cooperation between professionals but also the active and conscious participation of the patient, who is now seen as the protagonist of their healing process. The patient, having access to a wider range of therapeutic possibilities, can develop a deeper look at themselves, understanding their illnesses not only as isolated events or biological fatalities but as symbolic messages from their vibrational field, alerting to internal aspects that cry out for recognition, healing, and realignment. This integrative perspective allows treatment to go beyond mere symptom suppression, transforming into a real opportunity for personal growth and expansion of consciousness. From this vision, health is no longer understood as the mere absence of disease, but is understood as a dynamic state of harmony, where body, mind, and soul vibrate in tune with the greater purpose of each being and with the evolutionary forces that govern existence in its totality.

The synergy between Arcturian medicine and conventional medicine manifests naturally and harmoniously when both are understood not as competing or opposing forces, but as complementary within the same field of care and understanding of health. Conventional medicine, with its solid foundation in laboratory tests, biochemical analyses, sophisticated imaging techniques, and a wide range of diagnostic resources, offers the patient and healthcare professional a clear and quantifiable view of the body's physical state. This view, based on physiological parameters and concrete evidence, allows for the early detection of pathologies, monitoring of clinical evolution, and the application of targeted and effective interventions, especially in situations of urgency or imminent risk.

While conventional medicine unravels the physical and measurable signs of disease, Arcturian medicine expands this view beyond dense matter, entering the patient's vibrational, emotional, and spiritual field. Through refined intuitive perception,

Arcturian therapists are trained to directly access the being's energy field, identifying areas of blockage, stagnation, or fragmentation that do not appear in conventional exams but represent the vibrational roots of physical manifestations. This energetic reading is complemented by the channeling of information, where the patient's own higher consciousness—or that of related spiritual beings and guides—offers insights into the deep origin of the disharmony and the most appropriate paths for its resolution.

The analysis of the energy field allows for the detection not only of momentary blockages but also of recurring patterns that may have ancestral or transgenerational origins, often linked to past life memories or soul contracts signed in other existences. This hidden dimension of the disease is brought to consciousness so that the patient not only treats the symptom but understands the broader context of their condition, seeing the illness as a symbolic expression of internal processes that cry out for recognition and transformation. When the two approaches meet—the objective precision of medical science and the subtle breadth of Arcturian reading—an integrated and expanded view of health emerges, where the physical body is only the most visible layer of a multidimensional being in constant process of adjustment and learning.

This complementarity, however, is only fully realized when there is genuine collaboration between doctors and therapists, built on foundations of open dialogue, mutual respect, and recognition of the strengths and limitations of each system. This ideal collaboration involves periodic meetings, where information from clinical exams, laboratory results, and medical evaluations are cross-referenced with energetic readings and channelings obtained in the subtle field. This exchange does not aim to establish a hierarchy between knowledge, but to build a web of information that allows the patient to be understood in all their complexity. Clarity in communication between professionals ensures that no information is lost or interpreted in isolation, avoiding both the neglect of critical physical factors and the invalidation of subtle perceptions essential to the healing process.

The construction of individualized treatment plans emerges as a natural consequence of this integration. Instead of rigid protocols applied in a standardized way, each patient is seen as a unique combination of genetic, historical, emotional, spiritual, and environmental factors. This integrative vision allows each care plan to be carefully adjusted, contemplating both the necessary medications, surgical interventions, and conventional therapies, as well as the vibrational practices, directed meditations, emotional release techniques, and spiritual reconnection that support inner transformation. This personalization not only respects the uniqueness of the being, but also increases adherence to treatment, since the patient begins to recognize their active role in their own healing journey.

Case studies documenting this successful integration illustrate in concrete terms the power of this fusion. Patients diagnosed with cancer, for example, by combining conventional oncology treatments with Arcturian harmonization and vibrational reprogramming sessions, not only show a better response to medications and fewer side effects, but also report a new understanding of their life stories and a reframing of their own illness. In cases of autoimmune diseases, where conventional medicine is often limited to controlling symptoms with immunosuppressants, the Arcturian approach reveals deep emotional connections linked to memories of rejection or self-denial, allowing the patient to dissolve the patterns of self-attack that fuel the disordered immune response.

Similarly, patients with chronic pain, after years of pilgrimage through different medical specialties without definitive relief, find in the combination of conventional physiotherapy, analgesic medications, and energy realignment techniques a new way of understanding pain, often perceiving it as a voice of the body calling attention to areas of life where limits were not respected or emotions were repressed. In mental disorders such as anxiety and depression, the combination of psychiatric follow-up, traditional psychotherapy, and Arcturian harmonization allows access to deep unconscious layers, often linked to soul fragments disconnected in past traumas, promoting a psychic and spiritual reintegration that enhances the effectiveness of conventional treatments.

This integrative approach, by combining the precision of medical science with the depth of soul medicine, allows healing to be understood as a process that transcends the elimination of symptoms, involving a true inner transformation. Arcturian medicine, by illuminating the subtle roots of diseases and promoting reconnection with the being's spiritual essence, strengthens the patient's inner resilience and their ability to face the challenges of illness with awareness and dignity. In parallel, conventional medicine, by ensuring clinical stability, controlling the most aggressive symptoms, and preventing serious complications, creates a safe ground where vibrational healing can flourish without endangering the patient's physical integrity.

The full integration of these two medicines does not mean choosing between science or spirituality, but recognizing that both are complementary expressions of the same healing intelligence that permeates the universe. Each examination, each medication, each vibrational technique, or guided visualization thus becomes part of the same sacred field of care, where body, mind, and soul are honored as inseparable aspects of an evolving being. More than a set of techniques, this integration represents a new awareness of what it means to heal—not just to repair flaws or eliminate symptoms, but to restore the lost harmony between the being and their essential purpose, between their past experiences and their future potential, between their biology and their spirituality.

In practice, this fusion does not impose dogmas or exclusions. The patient is invited to occupy the center of their healing process, being heard in their beliefs, respected in their limits, and encouraged to express their preferences. The disease is no longer a sentence and becomes a journey—an opportunity to reconnect with oneself in all layers of being. Thus, each medical intervention is seen as a gesture of self-love, and each vibrational practice translates into concrete actions of self-care. Health, then, ceases to be merely the absence of disease and begins to be lived as a dynamic state of coherence, where body, mind, and soul vibrate in resonance with the essential truth of who one is and with the greater flow of life.

Thus, conventional medicine and Arcturian medicine, far from competing, intertwine in the same field of healing, where science and spirituality, reason and intuition, matter and energy merge to reveal the totality of the human being and the immense healing potential that emerges when body and soul speak the same language again.

In this encounter between science and spirituality, healing is no longer just the search for the extinction of a symptom and becomes a path of reconnection with the wholeness of being, where each examination, each medication, and each vibrational practice are understood as parts of the same sacred dialogue between the visible and the invisible. When doctors and therapists, science and ancestral wisdom, the patient and their own soul stand side by side in respect and cooperation, a fertile field is created where health flourishes not as a destination, but as a dynamic state of balance, presence, and alignment with the deepest purpose of existing.

Chapter 26
The Expansion of Consciousness and Planetary Healing

The evolution of individual consciousness presents itself as a continuous and integrated process, in which each human being perceives themselves as an inseparable extension of the planetary web of life. From the Arcturian perspective, this expansion does not occur in isolation or merely intellectually, but rather as a simultaneous awakening of the heart, mind, and soul, in which the individual progressively aligns with higher frequencies of love, compassion, and service to the common good. This expansive movement amplifies the perception of the self, dissolving the rigid barriers of the ego and allowing the human being to understand their active participation in the energetic and spiritual dynamics of the Earth. This expanded consciousness leads to the understanding that every thought, every emotion, and every intention emanates as a subtle vibration, intertwining with the collective field and shaping shared reality. The Arcturians understand that this conscious integration between the personal microcosm and the planetary macrocosm is the key to true global healing, where the restoration of external balance directly reflects the internal process of self-realization and harmonization of the being.

In this perspective, the path of expanding consciousness reveals itself as a journey of profound self-discovery, where the healing of ancestral traumas, limiting beliefs, and crystallized emotional patterns not only liberates the individual psyche, but also purifies and elevates the vibrational frequency of the energetic field around it. Each internal transformation reverberates in the subtle fabric of the Earth, contributing to the dissolution of collective patterns of fear, separation, and conflict. The Arcturians emphasize that planetary healing is not limited to external interventions in ecosystems or social systems, but emerges primarily from the internal purification of each being. By healing their own wounds, transmuting their shadows, and reconnecting with their divine essence, the individual becomes a conscious channel of universal light, radiating frequencies of harmony, compassion, and unity to the entire planet. This active role as co-creator of planetary reality is recognized as a spiritual commitment, where personal evolution and planetary regeneration intertwine as reflections of the same evolutionary flow.

Beyond personal healing, the Arcturian expansion of consciousness reinforces the importance of loving service to the collective as a natural expression of spiritual awakening. Recognizing that all beings are interconnected in a vast unified field of consciousness, the individual expands their compassion and sense of responsibility beyond their own needs and interests, actively integrating into initiatives that promote the common good. This conscious service is not restricted to specific acts of charity, but is permeated by the perception that every gesture, however small, carries the ability to sow vibrations of healing and balance throughout the planetary ecosystem. In this context, the practice of collective meditation, the creative visualization of a peaceful world, and the intentional transmission of healing energies are understood as spiritual technologies of high potency, capable of accelerating planetary regeneration and attuning humanity to the harmonic flows of the cosmos. By assuming their role as a conscious co-creator, the awakened human being aligns their existence with the greater purpose of serving as a bridge between matter and spirit, between the individual and the collective, between inner healing and global healing.

The understanding of the contribution of individual healing to planetary healing is based on the Arcturian view that the consciousness of each human being, in its vibrational essence, acts as a fundamental piece in the vast energetic mosaic of the planet. Every thought, every emotion nurtured in silence, and every action taken, even those seemingly insignificant, emanate subtle waves that intertwine with the collective field. This invisible, yet powerful, interconnection reveals that the process of inner healing does not remain restricted to the intimate space of the individual psyche, but reverberates and merges with the living web of the Earth. When a human being dedicates themselves to releasing deeply rooted negative patterns, dissolving ancestral traumas preserved for generations, and questioning limiting beliefs that have hardened their view of themselves and the world, this liberation not only relieves their soul, but also contributes to the purification of the planetary psychosphere. It is as if each layer of dissolved pain and each veil of illusion torn releases a portion of repressed light, which immediately reintegrates into the vibrational flow of the Earth, elevating, albeit subtly, the collective frequency of humanity.

As this expansion of individual consciousness advances, compassion, genuine empathy, and openness to unconditional love emerge as natural fruits — qualities that, when sprouting in the fertile soil of the awakened soul, expand the threads of connection between all beings. Empathy ceases to be just an emotional skill, becoming a direct perception of the essential unity that links every form of life. Compassion, in turn, arises from the deep understanding that the pain of another is never isolated, but echoes like a dissonant note in the entire planetary symphony. From this intimate perception emerges a new way of being in the world, in which the impulse to contribute to the collective well-being and to the healing of the Earth is no longer seen as a moral obligation or a forced act of altruism, but rather as the spontaneous expression of one's own spiritual identity.

It is in this perspective that the Arcturians emphasize, with crystal clarity, that true happiness and lasting well-being are not the result of the accumulation of goods or the fulfillment of personal desires disconnected from the whole. Authentic happiness arises from the generous flow of giving and receiving, of placing one's own talents, gifts, and unique abilities at the service of the collective, recognizing that personal destiny is intrinsically intertwined with the destiny of humanity and the planet. By extending one's hands to embrace the pain of another, offering a specific talent to collaborate on healing projects, or even consciously choosing words and thoughts that radiate harmony, each individual not only contributes to planetary regeneration, but also finds, in this expansive movement of surrender, the fulfillment of their own life purpose. This is the sacred paradox that the Arcturians teach: by stepping out of oneself and opening up to the whole, the individual returns to their deepest center, where their divine essence is revealed and where happiness ceases to be a search and becomes a natural condition of existence.

Within this flow of conscious expansion and service, the Arcturians offer a set of specific spiritual techniques to channel Arcturian energy for the benefit of peace and planetary harmony. These practices, when performed with pure intention and an open heart, transform into powerful tools of co-creation and vibrational alignment between humanity and the harmonic flows of the cosmos. Among these techniques, the practice of group meditation stands out, a spiritual technology that exponentially amplifies the power of collective intention. In this practice, groups of individuals gather, in person or remotely, with the common purpose of anchoring and radiating frequencies of peace, healing, and harmony to the Earth. The synergy between minds and hearts attuned to the same vibration creates a field of quantum coherence capable of crossing geographical boundaries and reaching vulnerable points of the planetary energy field, accelerating processes of purification and restoration.

In addition to meditation, the creative visualization of planetary healing is presented as another fundamental key to manifesting more harmonious realities. In this exercise, each participant is invited to construct, with richness of detail and genuine emotion, the mental image of a regenerated Earth — clear rivers meandering through green landscapes, forests vibrating in health and biodiversity, human communities living in harmony with each other and with nature, sustainable technologies integrated into natural cycles. This visualization, charged with loving intention, is not a simple mental fantasy, but rather a vibrational seed planted in the fertile soil of the quantum field, where potential realities await the creative impulse to manifest.

Another recommended practice is the direct transmission of healing energy to the planet, which can be carried out in different ways, adapted to the affinities of each individual. A simple technique consists of placing one's hands facing the Earth, in a meditative posture, and visualizing a golden or light blue light flowing from the center of the heart, down the arms, and radiating through the palms of the hands, enveloping the soil, oceans, forests, and all forms of life with this healing energy. Alternatively, this transmission can occur through telepathic connection with specific points on the planet — regions in conflict, areas of deforestation, or contaminated bodies of water — sending, with firmness and love, vibrational impulses of harmony, regeneration, and balance.

Finally, the Arcturians emphasize the importance of integrating this energetic service with concrete actions in the physical plane. Actively participating in volunteer projects in NGOs, environmental protection initiatives, or social programs that promote the well-being of vulnerable communities are ways of anchoring the subtle frequencies worked on the spiritual plane in the material world. True Arcturian service unites heaven and earth, spirit and matter, intention and action, creating an ascending spiral of transformation that involves all dimensions of existence.

By combining these practices — collective meditation, creative visualization, energy transmission, and active service — each individual becomes a conscious focal point of Arcturian energy, a living channel between the higher plane and earthly reality. More than isolated techniques, these practices integrate into a spiritualized lifestyle, in which every daily choice, every cultivated thought, and every gesture performed carries within it the intention to collaborate with planetary ascension. And so, in the harmonious intertwining between inner healing and global healing, the Earth rediscovers its path back to the light, guided by the hands and hearts of those who have chosen to serve as living bridges between matter and spirit.

In this constant intertwining between awakened consciousness and the living pulsation of the planet, the human being finally understands that their spiritual journey is inseparable from the collective journey of the Earth. Every step taken towards the inner light echoes in the pulse of planetary consciousness, like a single note that integrates into the greater melody of cosmic evolution. The Arcturians remind us that, by assuming this sacred responsibility, we become gardeners of a new reality, sowing, in the fertile soil of the present, the vibrations and intentions that will shape the common future. Planetary healing, therefore, is not a distant utopia, but a living and present process, woven in the silence of meditations, in the purity of intentions, and in the firmness of each act of conscious love. And so, the Earth and its children walk together, awakening each other, reminding each other of their stellar origin and their luminous destiny among the stars.

Chapter 27
The Ethics of Arcturian Medicine in Practice

The practice of Arcturian medicine is founded on an ethical code that transcends simple guidelines of conduct and is based on a deep understanding of the sacredness of each being and the interconnection between the subtle fields that permeate existence. Each Arcturian therapist is invited to recognize that, when accessing a patient's energy field, they are not only acting on an isolated individual, but are directly interacting with the planetary and cosmic energy web, in which all beings are intertwined. This awareness radically expands the notion of therapeutic responsibility, as each intervention, however small it may seem, reverberates beyond the personal sphere and affects the collective balance. The ethical commitment, in this context, is not limited to compliance with norms or protocols, but emerges from the non-negotiable perception that integrity, unrestricted respect for the spiritual sovereignty of the other, and purity of intention are structural elements of healing practice. Every therapeutic act is, therefore, an act of sacred service, in which the therapist becomes a channel of a superior and loving intelligence, never imposing their personal will, but acting in harmony with the guidance of Arcturian consciousness and with the natural flow of the patient's soul evolution.

Within this perspective, ethics in Arcturian medicine encompasses not only external conduct, but also the internal state of the therapist, who is constantly called to cultivate emotional clarity, mental neutrality, and vibrational purity so that their actions are free from ego interference, unconscious projections, or desires for personal recognition. Before each session, it is essential that the therapist harmonizes internally through practices of meditation, conscious breathing, and connection with their higher self, ensuring that they act as a transparent and unobstructed vehicle of Arcturian healing energy. This ethical inner alignment is considered as relevant as the technical application of practices, since the quality of the channeled energy directly reflects the state of consciousness of the one who directs it. This ethical commitment to one's own inner purification creates a field of trust and security that allows the patient to relax and open up to the therapeutic process, favoring a transparent and respectful interaction, where consent, boundaries, and confidentiality arise not as formal obligations, but as natural expressions of a relationship of deep mutual reverence.

Continuous deepening in the knowledge of Arcturian medicine is also understood as an essential part of the ethical commitment, since each therapist is encouraged to recognize themselves as an eternal learner, open to revisiting their beliefs, improving their skills, and expanding their understanding from new experiences and reflections. This posture of intellectual and spiritual humility avoids the crystallization of dogmas or authoritarian postures and keeps the therapist attuned to the dynamic fluidity of Arcturian wisdom, which is updated and refined as the collective consciousness of humanity evolves. This constant search for technical and ethical excellence does not occur in isolation, but is enriched by dialogue and the exchange of experiences with other therapists, by participation in study circles and collective meditation, and by the cultivation of an attitude of selfless and compassionate service. In this way, Arcturian medicine manifests itself not only as a therapeutic system, but as a true school of ethical and spiritual evolution, where each therapist, in healing, also heals themselves, and in serving, also aligns with their own divine essence, becoming a beacon of integrity, love, and wisdom in the midst of the great planetary transition in progress.

The importance of ethics and responsibility in the practice of Arcturian medicine manifests itself, first and foremost, in the deep awareness that manipulating or acting on the subtle fields of a being is not a trivial action or one devoid of consequences. Every energetic movement, every directed intention, and every frequency emitted during a therapeutic session can reverberate in unexpected ways, crossing layers of the patient's spiritual and emotional structure and, in many cases, projecting beyond them, reaching the collective energy networks and ancestral links that connect them to their cosmic and earthly lineages. In this scenario, acting ethically means understanding that the role of the Arcturian therapist is not that of a performer of techniques or a manipulator of energy flows, but that of a careful guardian of the harmony that sustains the internal balance of the patient and the larger web in which that being is inserted. The pure intention of healing, devoid of egoic desires, therapeutic ambitions, or the craving for quick results, becomes a non-negotiable foundation. This purity of purpose is what aligns the therapist with the higher Arcturian frequencies, allowing the healing energy to manifest in its most crystalline and respectful state.

Arcturian ethics, therefore, embraces deep respect for the limits and sovereignty of the being being treated, recognizing that each soul has its own evolutionary rhythm, its layers of protection, and its learning processes, which should not be violated or hastened under any circumstances. This respect is expressed not only in external conduct, but also in the vibrational posture and internal calibration of the therapist, who learns to sustain the therapeutic space without invading or projecting their own expectations or beliefs onto it. Every technique, every emission of light or sound, every subtle touch applied during a session must spring from this absolute reverence for the patient's integrity, never crossing the boundaries that their soul has chosen to preserve.

Ethical responsibility is also manifested in the continuous search for professional excellence and expansion of knowledge. Arcturian medicine, being a living and adaptable science, does not crystallize into fixed dogmas or immutable scripts. Each therapist is called to recognize themselves as a perpetual learner, willing to revisit their understandings, test their approaches, and integrate new perspectives as their sensitivity and connection with higher consciousnesses deepen. This constant updating occurs through multiple paths: the reading of specialized literature, where the reports of more experienced therapists offer valuable clues about vibrational traps, technical variations, and ways to refine sensitivity; participation in workshops and immersive courses, which offer not only theoretical content, but also the direct experience of expanded states of consciousness, the refinement of energetic perception, and the exercise of subtle listening.

These learning encounters also function as spaces for exchange between therapists, in which experiences are shared and analyzed together, allowing mistakes and successes to be converted into collective wisdom. It is in this environment of humility and constant exchange that Arcturian medicine flourishes, free from the isolation of the solitary therapist and sustained by an egregore of continuous learning, where each healer is called to offer their unique perception and to welcome the visions and contributions of others.

However, Arcturian ethics is not limited to technical improvement and the exchange of experiences. It also includes a personal commitment to one's own vibrational purification. Before any service, the therapist is guided to perform a process of inner harmonization, preparing their energy field to act as a pure channel of

Arcturian consciousness. This preparation involves a careful sequence of steps:

First, it is recommended that the therapist retreat to a quiet space, where they can disconnect from daily activities and stimuli. There, sitting in a comfortable position, they begin a cycle of conscious breathing, with long, deep inhalations, followed by gentle exhalations, allowing each exhalation to release accumulated physical, emotional, and mental tensions. Then, with their eyes closed, the therapist visualizes a column of golden light descending from the galactic center to the top of their head, penetrating through the crown chakra and slowly running down their entire spine, filling each cell with this living and conscious light.

With the mind quieted and the body relaxed, the therapist then invokes the presence of their Higher Self and Arcturian consciousness, declaring in voice or thought their intention to act only as a pure and transparent channel of healing energy, without interference from the ego, the mind, or unconscious conditioning. This declaration of intention is considered a sacred commitment and functions as a vibrational seal that protects the therapeutic field from external and internal interference.

After this initial connection, the therapist performs a quick scan of their own energy field, identifying and dissolving tensions or emotional patterns that may be vibrating in their system. This self-cleaning is essential, as the energy channeled during the session always crosses the therapist's field, and any residue or personal distortion can contaminate the purity of the

Arcturian flow. Only after this preparation is the therapist considered ready to receive the patient and open the therapeutic space.

This ethical care with one's own vibrational state is not an optional detail, but an essential part of the therapist's responsibility. By taking care of themselves, they take care of the patient. By purifying their intention, they preserve the sacredness of the healing process. This perception naturally unfolds in the way consent, confidentiality, and professional boundaries are treated in Arcturian medicine.

From the first contact, the therapist is instructed to establish a clear and loving communication with the patient, explaining in a simple and accessible way what Arcturian medicine is, which techniques can be applied, what sensations the patient may experience, and what are the benefits and eventual transient discomforts of the process. This initial dialogue creates a field of trust, where informed consent emerges as a natural act of mutual respect and not as a bureaucratic formality.

Confidentiality, in turn, is understood as the integral preservation of the privacy and sacredness of the experiences shared during the session. The Arcturian therapist is called to listen with full presence and to keep every word, every emotion, and every revelation as one who cares for a divine secret, understanding that there, in that space of sacred listening, the patient's soul is revealing itself in its deepest vulnerability.

Professional boundaries, as important as the other layers of Arcturian ethics, arise from the recognition that the therapist is not the savior or the master of the one seeking help. Defining and sustaining these boundaries – both in the physical space of the session and on the emotional and spiritual levels – ensures that the patient's autonomy is preserved and that the therapist does not overstep the role of facilitator to assume control or responsibility for the other's healing process.

Thus, the ethical and responsible practice of Arcturian medicine is not just a set of external guidelines, but a way of living one's own spirituality in the therapeutic act, where every gesture is impregnated with reverence and every word is spoken from the heart. By maintaining this commitment to purity and respect, the therapist creates a safe, loving, and welcoming field, where true healing can flourish – one that is not imposed from the outside in, but that gently sprouts from the soul that, feeling seen, recognized, and honored, remembers its own light and allows itself to shine.

In this continuous ethical refinement, the Arcturian therapist recognizes that their own presence is, in itself, part of the medicine they offer. More than the techniques applied or the energies channeled, it is the vibrational quality of their consciousness — nourished by humility, reverence, and unconditional love — that establishes the true space of healing. Each therapeutic encounter, therefore, transcends the functional character of a session and transforms into a sacred ritual, where two fields of consciousness intertwine in search of harmonization and awakening. In this space of mutual respect, the therapist does not place themselves above or in front, but alongside, as a silent presence that holds the torch of light just enough for the patient to see the next step of their journey. And it is in this delicate flow, where ethics and spirituality become inseparable, that Arcturian medicine reveals its true essence: a path of healing that respects the sacredness of each soul and honors, in every gesture, the divine pulse that unites all beings in the great cosmic organism of existence.

Chapter 28
The Training of Arcturian Therapists

The training of Arcturian therapists, imbued with ancient wisdom and subtle energies, transcends the acquisition of technical knowledge, delving into the understanding of the interconnection between intuition, energy, and consciousness. The Arcturian civilization, with its profound knowledge of the nature of healing, establishes clear guidelines for the training of Arcturian therapists. The Arcturian approach is based on the development of intuition, the practice of meditation and visualization, and the pursuit of self-knowledge.

The development of intuition, fundamental in the training of Arcturian therapists, involves the practice of meditation, mindfulness, and connection with inner wisdom. Meditation helps to quiet the mind, expand consciousness, and open the channels of intuition. Mindfulness, the careful observation of bodily sensations, emotions, and thoughts, helps to perceive the subtle signs of intuition. The connection with inner wisdom, the search for self-knowledge and reflection on life experiences, helps to develop confidence in intuition and improve the ability to discern.

The practice of meditation and visualization, pillars of Arcturian therapist training, helps to strengthen the connection with universal energy, develop the ability to channel healing energy, and enhance creative visualization. Meditation, the regular practice of quieting the mind and connecting with inner peace, helps to strengthen the connection with universal energy and expand consciousness. Visualization, the practice of creating vivid and detailed mental images, helps to develop the ability to direct healing energy and enhance creative visualization, essential for the practice of psychic surgery and distance healing.

The pursuit of self-knowledge, essential in the training of Arcturian therapists, manifests as a constant call for inner observation and the journey towards one's own essence, recognizing in each fold of the soul a reflection of one's greater mission. This process, far from being merely reflective or philosophical, is experienced as a deep dive into the waters of consciousness, where each layer of beliefs, fears, and conditioning is gradually revealed and, upon being embraced, transmuted. Self-observation becomes, in this context, a daily practice, almost like a spiritual breath, in which the therapist in training learns to map their instinctive reactions, emotional responses, and automatic thought flows that shape their view of themselves and the world. It is not enough to identify superficial patterns — the Arcturian gaze is trained to penetrate the essence, unveiling the hidden layers where unhealed wounds still echo in the form of distorted self-image or limiting beliefs.

This self-observation is accompanied by a constant exercise of deep reflection on the values and beliefs that guide the therapist's journey. More than simple records or mental reviews, this reflection takes the form of internal dialogues in which each value, each conviction, is subjected to the light of higher consciousness. Why do we believe what we believe? What is the origin of each value that guides us? Are we based on an internal truth, or do we reproduce cultural, family, or spiritual inheritances that no longer match the voice of our soul? This continuous questioning is part of the Arcturian training, because only those who recognize the roots of their own belief system can act as a clean channel, without projections or distortions, for the healing energy that flows through their presence.

In parallel with this attentive look at beliefs and values, Arcturian training encourages the courage to explore the less illuminated territories of one's own being — the traumas and negative behavior patterns that, hidden or repressed, continue to act as silent forces that sabotage inner growth and the clarity of the energy channel. This exploration is not a casual or superficial act; it requires surrender and willingness to revisit buried memories, forgotten pains, and unconscious pacts that continue to fuel cycles of repetition. This journey can be made through specific meditative practices, where the therapist is guided to revisit key moments in their history, not only as an observer, but as a conscious participant, capable of rewriting, reframing, and, finally, releasing what no longer serves their evolutionary journey.

In many cases, external therapeutic support is not only recommended, but valued as part of the training.

Working with other Arcturian therapists, or with therapists of complementary approaches, allows the future therapist to experience the patient's position, consciously making themselves vulnerable to understand, firsthand, the processes of acceptance, healing, and reintegration. This direct experience expands empathy and offers practical learning on how to create safe and compassionate spaces for those who, in the future, will seek their assistance.

This inner dive, however, does not end with the release of traumas or the deconstruction of beliefs. It expands into an even vaster territory: the search for life purpose. For the Arcturians, there is no true healing without alignment with the soul's purpose — that intimate calling that connects the individual being to the greater flow of creation. Finding this purpose is not a linear task, but a progressive unfolding of inner listening, sincere surrender, and willingness to serve. The therapist is guided to investigate which gifts and talents already emerge naturally from their essence, and how these gifts can be offered to the world as authentic expressions of their inner truth.

To facilitate this alignment, the training includes regular practices of connection with the divine essence — that sacred spark that inhabits the heart of every being and holds the memories of the soul's original path. These practices may include specific meditations to tune into personal Akashic records, where the therapist learns to access information about their past lives, previous choices, and spiritual commitments made before their current incarnation. This process of reconnecting with divine purpose is gradual and respects the unique rhythm of each soul, but it is always supported by the understanding that an Arcturian therapist can only truly lead another being to meet their essence if they themselves have already walked through this inner territory with humility and courage.

Integrating this dimension of self-knowledge with theoretical and practical knowledge is another fundamental pillar of Arcturian training. The study of energetic anatomy, for example, is not approached as a simple memorization of structures or functions, but as a living map that reveals and transforms itself as the therapist delves into the understanding of their own subtle anatomy. Each chakra, each meridian, each energetic body is felt internally, experienced in daily practices, and understood as a direct reflection of the therapist's own state of consciousness and inner balance. Thus, when studying the human energy field, the Arcturian therapist not only accumulates technical knowledge, but recognizes in each point, in each flow, and in each blockage a direct resonance with their own journey.

The same occurs in the learning of Arcturian healing techniques, which include laying on of hands, energetic acupuncture, psychic surgery, and distance healing. Each technique is practiced first on the therapist themselves, allowing them to feel, firsthand, how each intervention affects the subtle flows of energy, and how the intention, mental clarity, and emotional purity of the channel directly interfere with the effectiveness of the process. In this way, the practice does not become a mechanical act, but a living expression of the healing consciousness that the therapist develops within themselves.

Professional ethics and understanding of current legislation are equally incorporated as part of this process of self-knowledge and inner alignment. For the Arcturians, ethics is not just a set of external rules, but a natural manifestation of the therapist's inner integrity. Informed consent, confidentiality, and legal responsibility are seen as direct extensions of respect and reverence for the sacred journey of each being. Thus, ethical practice is not born from fear of punishment or the desire for conformity, but from the deep awareness that each therapeutic act is a co-creation between souls, where mutual respect and clarity of intentions are essential for true healing to manifest.

Finally, Arcturian training is completed with participation in internships and mentorships, where theoretical knowledge and inner development find their field of practical application. During internships, the therapist in training observes, accompanies, and gradually assumes the conduct of sessions under the direct supervision of experienced therapists. This practical experience allows not only technical refinement, but also the development of therapeutic presence — that subtle quality that transforms each encounter into a safe and luminous space of healing.

Mentorships, in turn, offer an intimate space for reflection and improvement, where the therapist in training can share their doubts, challenges, and discoveries with a mentor who has already walked this path. This bond of trust allows the future therapist to receive precious feedback, adjusting their practices and deepening their self-knowledge in light of the experience of someone who has already integrated, within themselves, knowing and being. Thus, the training of Arcturian therapists is revealed not only as a technical learning, but as a living journey of self-discovery, healing, and reconnection with the greater purpose of serving the light of universal consciousness.

At the end of this formative journey, the Arcturian therapist understands that their true diploma is not conferred by an external institution, but by the very pulse of their soul, which recognizes in their path of self-transformation the necessary preparation to welcome, without judgment or projections, the pain and light of each being that will seek their help. Each technique learned, each practice perfected, and each theory assimilated only comes to life when it passes through the filter of personal experience, becoming embodied wisdom — a knowing that flows not from the isolated mind, but from the awakened heart, where compassion and clarity walk side by side. Thus, Arcturian training does not end a cycle, but inaugurates a new stage of conscious service, where the therapist recognizes themselves as an eternal learner and humble guardian of an ancestral legacy that, at each session, is reborn in the sacred encounter between two souls in search of healing and truth.

Chapter 29
The Future of Arcturian Medicine

The future of Arcturian medicine unfolds as a dynamic horizon where science and spirituality cease to occupy opposite poles and merge into an evolutionary synergy, allowing healing to transcend the limitations of matter and reach the subtle layers of human existence. This medicine of the future is not restricted to the treatment of isolated symptoms, but understands the human being as a multidimensional field in constant interaction with its physical, energetic, and cosmic environment. In this new therapeutic era, each individual is recognized as a vibrational being whose health depends on the balance between their emotions, thoughts, life purpose, and their connection with the universal forces that sustain life throughout the cosmos. Arcturian medicine therefore advances towards a model of integral care in which cutting-edge technology, intuitive sensitivity, and ancestral practices act in an integrated way, promoting not only healing but the awakening of consciousness and the reconnection of the human being with their co-creative role in the web of planetary life.

The improvement of Arcturian vibrational technologies represents one of the pillars of this expanded medicine, where resonant frequency devices are capable of mapping energetic imbalances in the subtle fields and correcting dissonant patterns before they crystallize in the physical body. Quantum biofeedback equipment, cell regeneration chambers based on sacred geometries, and therapeutic holography systems allow the patient's energy field to be harmonized in real time, promoting a complete vibrational reconfiguration. However, these technologies are understood not as substitutes for human consciousness, but as sophisticated extensions of the therapist's intuitive perception, who remains the main channel of connection between higher wisdom and the patient's reality. In this new approach, the Arcturian therapist is trained to work in partnership with highly sensitive artificial intelligences, which cross-reference vibrational data, life histories, and multidimensional information, offering precious insights to personalize therapeutic approaches that respect the unique path of each soul.

The strengthening of intuition as a clinical tool is another fundamental axis in the Arcturian medicine of the future. Therapists not only develop their perceptive abilities to feel energy flows or visualize subtle fields, but are encouraged to cultivate empathic telepathy and direct listening to the higher layers of consciousness, where the deepest information about each patient's history, mission, and spiritual challenges resides. Innovative protocols integrate conscious channeling practices into the therapeutic process, allowing the therapist to access direct guidance from the patient's own higher consciousness, from the Arcturian spheres, or from Akashic fields, increasing the accuracy and depth of diagnoses. These practices, conducted with ethical rigor and deep respect for the patient's sovereignty, restore intuition to its central place in the art of healing, rescuing the ancestral wisdom that true health arises from harmony between the being and its divine purpose, and not only from the absence of symptoms.

The patient's autonomy, in this context, expands beyond simple informed decision-making, transforming itself into a continuous process of self-education, self-knowledge, and self-transformation. The Arcturian medicine of the future trains not only skilled therapists, but also entire communities of conscious beings, who understand their health as a direct reflection of their thoughts, emotions, and daily choices. Energy monitoring apps, interactive learning platforms, and spiritual support networks become tools accessible to everyone, offering not only technical information about their state of health, but also daily practices for vibrational elevation, guided meditations, and guidance for the co-creation of more harmonious personal and collective realities. In this way, the future of Arcturian medicine reveals itself as a collective evolutionary path, where each being, by taking care of themselves, actively collaborates for planetary regeneration and for the manifestation of an awakened, integrated humanity, vibrationally attuned to universal harmony.

The integration of advanced technologies in Arcturian medicine, an essential step towards the realization of this new therapeutic era, manifests itself in a comprehensive way and deeply connected to the frequencies that permeate the subtle and physical bodies of patients. This process involves the creation and constant evolution of healing devices based on specific vibrational frequencies, carefully calibrated to act on individual and collective energy fields. Among these technologies, harmonic resonance platforms and sophisticated light therapy systems stand out, in which beams of coded light, adjusted according to the vibrational needs of each being, gently penetrate the subtle bodies, realigning energy flows, dissolving crystallized blockages, and activating regenerative processes at cellular levels. This spectrum of action allows not only to restore the balance of organs and tissues, but to harmonize emotional and mental circuits that, at times, are the true roots of the dysfunctions manifested in the physical plane.

With the advancement of these technologies, the application of highly sensitive artificial intelligence also emerges, developed to interpret vast volumes of multidimensional information in real time. These platforms are not limited to crossing conventional biological data, but integrate information captured from the Akashic records, the vibrational signatures emitted by each cell, and the emotional and mental patterns recorded in the patient's subtle fields. By combining these elements, artificial intelligence offers a panoramic and deep view of the being, identifying not only emerging imbalances, but also their probable origins, karmic correlations, and potential personalized therapeutic paths. This predictive analysis capability allows the therapist, acting in harmony with these tools, to anticipate possible disharmonies before they materialize in the physical body, guiding the patient through a preventive process of healing and reconnection with themselves.

Within this technological spectrum, the creation of immersive virtual environments emerges as a natural extension of Arcturian therapeutic practices. Through virtual and augmented reality technologies, patients are guided to vibrational spaces tailored to their specific needs. These digital environments, far from being mere simulations, function as true resonance fields, where sacred geometries, sound frequencies, and light projections interact to reconfigure disharmonious vibrations and stimulate the restoration of inner harmony. In these spaces, the patient can walk through coded vibrational landscapes, immerse themselves in healing holograms that adjust their energy matrix, and participate in guided meditations where, through total immersion, they reconnect with their subtler layers and receive directly, in their conscious field, guidance and messages from their own higher essence.

This fusion of technology and spirituality, however, never neglects the central role of intuition as the sacred compass of therapeutic practice. The rescue of intuition, understood not as an esoteric gift reserved for a few, but as a natural ability accessible to all who are willing to cultivate it, is an essential pillar of the Arcturian medicine of the future. The development of specific techniques for refining energetic perception is encouraged from the early stages of therapist training, but is also made available to patients and communities, allowing everyone to, at some level, fine-tune their sensitivity and act as co-creators of their own health.

Among these techniques, continuous training in deep meditation stands out, where the practitioner learns to expand their perception beyond the physical body, capturing energy flows, subtle changes in vibrational fields, and information coded in their own aura. The constant practice of mindfulness, or conscious presence, strengthens this sensitivity, allowing the therapist or patient to perceive energetic variations associated with emotions, recurring thoughts, or external patterns of influence. This heightened perception allows not only to detect blockages or energetic invasions, but also to direct healing flows with precision, harmonizing subtle fields before disharmonies consolidate into physical symptoms.

In addition to expanded sensory perception, the practice of telepathy and clairaudience plays a prominent role in the integration of intuition into Arcturian medicine. Specific exercises are developed to stimulate telepathic communication, initially in pairs, where therapist and patient learn to establish direct channels of vibrational exchange, without the need for spoken words. Gradually, this process expands to the reception of information directly from the higher layers of the patient's own consciousness or from their spiritual mentors. Intuitive listening, or clairaudience, is refined through daily practices of inner silence, where the therapist learns to distinguish the subtle voice of inner wisdom from the noises of the conditioned mind, ensuring that the guidance received during the therapeutic process is always aligned with the patient's highest good.

To ensure that this integration of intuition into clinical practice occurs in a structured and safe manner, specific protocols are created to guide the conduct of channeling sessions and the use of intuitive questionnaires. These questionnaires, tailored to each patient, combine traditional questions with spaces for the therapist's intuitive insights, creating a dynamic overview where objective data and subtle perceptions complement each other. Conscious channeling sessions, conducted in a protected and vibrationally prepared environment, allow information from the Akashic records, higher consciousnesses, or even the patient's own higher self to be directly incorporated into the therapeutic process, enriching diagnoses and guiding therapeutic choices with precision and respect for the spiritual sovereignty of each being.

This strengthening of intuition goes hand in hand with the active promotion of patient autonomy, a core value in Arcturian medicine, which understands health as a direct reflection of consciousness and the individual responsibility of each being for their own evolutionary path. Health education, in this context, is not limited to the transmission of technical information about the functioning of the physical body, but includes the understanding of the multidimensional nature of the being and its continuous interaction with the collective field. Courses and lectures are offered on a regular basis, covering topics ranging from vibrational nutrition and energetic hygiene to advanced practices of self-connection and conscious cellular reprogramming. Informative materials, both printed and digital, are made available on multiple platforms, offering practical tools for each individual to understand their health as a direct reflection of their thoughts, emotions, choices, and spiritual alignment.

To support this journey of self-knowledge, energy monitoring apps are developed that go beyond simply measuring physical parameters such as blood pressure or heart rate. Quantum sensors integrated into these devices capture variations in the user's subtle fields, providing real-time feedback on the vibrational coherence of their thoughts and emotions. These apps, interconnected with educational platforms, suggest personalized daily harmonization practices, such as guided meditations, breathing exercises, specific mantras, or adjustments to the diet, promoting not only punctual healing, but the maintenance of a high and continuous vibrational state.

Finally, the creation of online support communities weaves a vibrational support network, where patients, therapists, and mentors share experiences, exchange insights, and strengthen bonds of belonging. Discussion forums address topics ranging from practical everyday issues to philosophical reflections on the role of humanity in planetary ascension. Collective meditation groups, led by experienced facilitators, generate fields of group coherence that amplify the connection with higher spheres and accelerate individual processes of healing and awakening. Regular group therapy sessions, held both in virtual and face-to-face environments, offer safe spaces for emotional expression, the exchange of knowledge, and the co-creation of new realities, where individual and collective healing intertwine as inseparable expressions of the same cosmic dance.

In this ever-expanding horizon, the Arcturian medicine of the future reveals itself as an invitation for humanity to remember its own co-creative nature, assuming not only responsibility for its physical and emotional health, but also for its spiritual harmony and its vibrational impact on the collective field. The Arcturian therapist, far from occupying the role of savior or exclusive holder of knowledge, becomes a guardian of consciousness, a loving facilitator who, by illuminating paths, reminds each human being of their innate capacity to access their own source of healing and wisdom. Thus, science and spirituality, technology and intuition, individual and collective intertwine in a sacred dance of healing, where the balance of the Earth and its inhabitants arises from the simple, yet profound, remembrance that all true healing is, above all, a return to one's own essence.

Epilogue

Upon crossing the final pages of this work, it is not merely a cycle of reading that comes to a close. What now pulsates in your hands and reverberates in your mind and soul is the seed of a new understanding—not only about healing, but about your own role in the great cosmic concert of existence. This book, with its revelations and practices, its reflections and invitations, does not end here. It is a point of ignition, an initial breath that now echoes in every cell of your body, in every thought you choose to nurture, and in every connection you remember with the invisible flows of life.

Throughout the pages, you were invited to realize that health and healing are infinitely vaster movements than the relief of symptoms or the search for immediate solutions. True healing is a journey. A gradual return to the natural state of harmony that your soul has always known, but that the modern mind has learned to forget. In each energetic practice, in each concept about the chakras, about the subtle flows, and about the interconnection between mind, body, and spirit, you did not just receive information. You received a calling—to feel, to listen, to remember.

And this remembering is the key to the entire path.

Arcturian integrative medicine, with its vibrational sophistication and cosmic tenderness, offers us a lens to see the invisible. To perceive how each accumulated emotion, each crystallized belief, each recurring thought silently sculpts the contours of our physical and spiritual health. More than techniques or knowledge, you have received throughout these pages a new perspective. A perspective that goes beyond the body as a machine and reaches the being as a living score of frequencies in constant dialogue with the universe.

This invitation to reconnection does not end here. In fact, it is just beginning. For the true integration of this knowledge does not happen in the intellect, but in everyday life. In the small choices. In the way you breathe, how you nourish yourself, how you silence yourself to listen to your own body, and how you welcome each emotion that crosses your chest. Healing, as the Arcturians reveal and as the ancestors of the Earth echo, is not a one-time event, but a state of continuous presence. It is the way you inhabit your own body-temple. How you care for your energy as one who cares for a sacred flame, knowing that every thought, every word, and every gesture are vibrational codes that weave your biological, emotional, and spiritual destiny.

By integrating this knowledge, you are no longer the same being who opened this book for the first time. Something has changed. Perhaps imperceptible to the hurried mind, but deeply recognized by the soul. You begin to perceive your own energy field as a living reality, capable of dialoguing with nature, with other beings, and with the cosmos itself. You perceive yourself as a bridge—between the visible and the invisible, between the body and the spirit, between the Earth and the stars.

This perception is the beginning of true spiritual and therapeutic autonomy. For being healthy, in this new paradigm, does not mean only the absence of symptoms, but full presence. Presence in your choices, in your cycles, in your connections, and in the way you choose to integrate the cosmic flow that runs through every cell of your body. Arcturian medicine is not just a healing system—it is a way of life. Of remembering that you are a moving field of light, a fractal of the Whole, dancing your uniqueness within the vastness of the cosmos.

And it is here, in this moment of closure and restart, that the true invitation is revealed. Because, upon finishing this reading, you are being called to become the guardian of your own journey. No one else holds the key to your health and your spiritual expansion. No technique, however advanced, replaces your own inner listening. No practice, however sophisticated it may seem, is more powerful than the conscious decision to return, day after day, to the simplicity of your essential being.

Every time you breathe consciously, every time you place your hands on your own heart and listen to what it has to say, every time you align yourself with nature, with the sunlight, with the silence of the stars, or with the wisdom of crystals, you are activating your own inner medicine. This is the greatest lesson left by the Arcturians and the ancestral traditions that echo in this work: true healing is not an external intervention, but an internal awakening. A reminder that your essence is already whole, complete, and vibrant. What you call healing is, in fact, just the unveiling of this forgotten truth.

May you, upon closing this book, not close the portal that has been opened within you. May each practice and each reflection reverberate not as distant theories, but as seeds planted in your own vibrational field. And may these seeds, nurtured by your attentive gaze and your open heart, blossom as a new way of inhabiting your body and your soul.

You do not walk alone. Not now, not ever. The invisible hands of Arcturian wisdom continue to touch your subtle field, guiding your steps with tenderness and precision. With each conscious breath, you are reminded: healing is not distant, it is the very path you walk with courage and presence. And each step, however small it may seem, is a celebration of the reunion with your luminous essence.

May this be only the beginning of your journey. May the horizon of healing expand with each new day, with each choice to live with presence, reverence, and love. And may you, upon recognizing your light, inspire others to remember their own. For, as the Arcturians whisper between the lines of time, the healing of one is the healing music of all.

www.ingramcontent.com/pod-product-compliance
Lightning Source LLC
LaVergne TN
LVHW040045080526
838202LV00045B/3493